Mediterranean Diet

Delectable Journey into Healthy Eating

Indulge in the Flavors of the Mediterranean Diet for Vibrant Health and Delicious Delights!

Jennifer Phillips

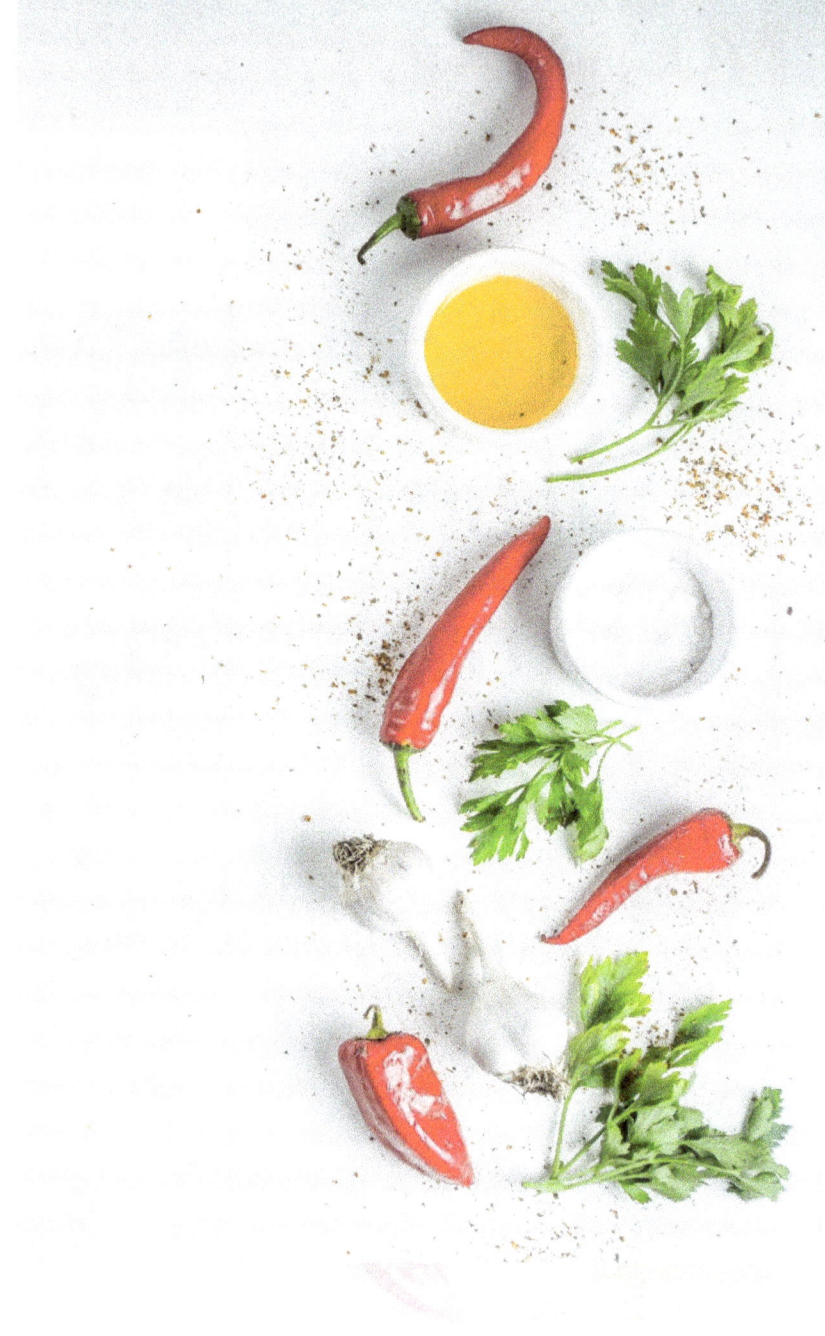

© Copyright 2023 by **Jennifer Phillips**- All rights reserved.

The following Book is reproduced below with the goal of providing information that is as accurate and reliable as possible. Regardless, purchasing this Book can be seen as consent to the fact that both the publisher and the author of this book are in no way experts on the topics discussed within and that any recommendations or suggestions that are made herein are for entertainment purposes only. Professionals should be consulted as needed prior to undertaking any of the action endorsed herein.

This declaration is deemed fair and valid by both the American Bar Association and the Committee of Publishers Association and is legally binding throughout the United States.

Furthermore, the transmission, duplication, or reproduction of any of the following work including specific information will be considered an illegal act irrespective of if it is done electronically or in print. This extends to creating a secondary or tertiary copy of the work or a recorded copy and is only allowed with the express written consent from the Publisher. All additional right reserved.

The information in the following pages is broadly considered a truthful and accurate account of facts and as such, any inattention, use, or misuse of the information in question by the reader will render any resulting actions solely under their purview. There are no scenarios in which the publisher or the original author of this work can be in any fashion deemed liable for any hardship or damages that may befall them after undertaking information described herein.

Additionally, the information in the following pages is intended only for informational purposes and should thus be thought of as universal. As befitting its nature, it is presented without assurance regarding its prolonged validity or interim quality. Trademarks that are mentioned are done without written consent and can in no way be considered an endorsement from the trademark holder.

All picture are under licence by CC BY-SA-NC and CC BY-NC

Table of content

MEDITERRANEAN BREAKFAST RECIPE 7
MULTIGRAIN TOAST WITH GRILLED VEGETABLES 8
Energizing Breakfast Protein Bars 10
Fruity Nutty Muesli 12
Egg Veggie Scramble 13
STRAPATSATHA 16
MEDITERRANEAN LUNCH RECIPE 18
Slow-Cooker Mediterranean Stew 19
Greek Cauliflower Rice Bowls with Grilled Chicken 22
Prosciutto Pizza with Corn & Arugula 24
Cheesy Spinach-&-Artichoke Stuffed Spaghetti Squash 26
Vegan Mediterranean Lentil Soup 28
EatingWell's Eggplant Parmesan 30
BBQ Shrimp with Garlicky Kale & Parmesan-Herb Couscous 32
MEDITERRANEAN SALAD RECIPES 34
LAHANOSALATA (CABBAGE SALAD) 35
TARAMOSALATA/TARAMA (FISH ROE SALAD) 36
GRILLED HALLOUMI SALAD 38
MEDITERRANEAN POULTRY RECIPES 40
CHICKEN GALANTINE 41
SPICY TURKEY BREAST WITH FRUIT CHUTNEY 43
GRILLED DUCK BREAST WITH FRUIT SALSA 45
QUAIL WITH PLUM SAUCE 46
MEDITERRANEAN SEAFOOD RECIPES 48
STEAMED SEAFOOD DINNER 49

GRILLED FISH WITH POLENTA 51
BACCALÁ 53
FLOUNDER WITH BALSAMIC REDUCTION 54
MEDITERRANEAN MEAT, BEEF AND PORK RECIPES 55
AUBERGINE MEAT ROLLS 56
PORK WITH LEEKS AND CELERY 59
STIFADO (BRAISED BEEF WITH ONIONS) 60
BRAISED LAMB SHOULDER 61
VEGETARIAN AND LEGUMES MEDITERRANEAN RECIPES 62
KIDNEY BEAN CASSEROLE 63
LENTIL AND WALNUT CHILI 64
RED LENTIL LASAGNA 65
GRILLED PORTOBELLO MUSHROOMS 66
MEDITERRANEAN DESSERTS 67
FRESH FRUIT AND MERINGUE 68
POACHED APPLES 69
CINNAMON ALMOND CAKE 71
Decorated Figs 72
MEDITERRANEAN BREAD 73
PASTOURMA PIE 74
PRASSOPITA (LEEK PIE) 77
MEDITERRANEAN RICE AND GRAINS 79
Low Sodium Garlic Parmesan Popcorn 80
MEDITERRANEAN EGG AND RECIPIES 82
Mediterranean Egg Mug 83
MEDITERRANEAN BREAKFAST BAKE 85

Texas Traditional Okra Bread 86
Gratitude Herb Bread 88
Asian Kale Bread 91
Tomato Sauce Bread 94
MEDITERRANEAN APPETIZERS 96
Mediterranean Nachos 97
Roasted Beet Muhammara 99

MEDITERRANEAN BREAKFAST RECIPE

MULTIGRAIN TOAST WITH GRILLED VEGETABLES

Serves 6

- 1/2 eggplant
- 1/2 zucchini
- 1/2 yellow squash
- 1/2 red pepper
- 1/2 yellow pepper
- 1/2 green pepper
- 1 teaspoon extra-virgin olive oil
- 6 multigrain bread slices
- 3 ounces goat cheese
- 1/4 bunch fresh marjoram Fresh-cracked black pepper, to taste

Directions

- Slice the eggplant, zucchini, and squash in 3-inch lengths, 1/4- to 1/2-inch thick, and cut the peppers in half. Preheat a grill to medium heat. Brush the vegetables with the oil and grill all until fork-tender. Cut all the vegetables into large dice. (Vegetables can be prepared the night before; refrigerate and reheat or bring to room temperature before serving.)
- Grill the bread until lightly toasted, then remove from heat and top with vegetables. Sprinkle with cheese, chopped marjoram, and black pepper.

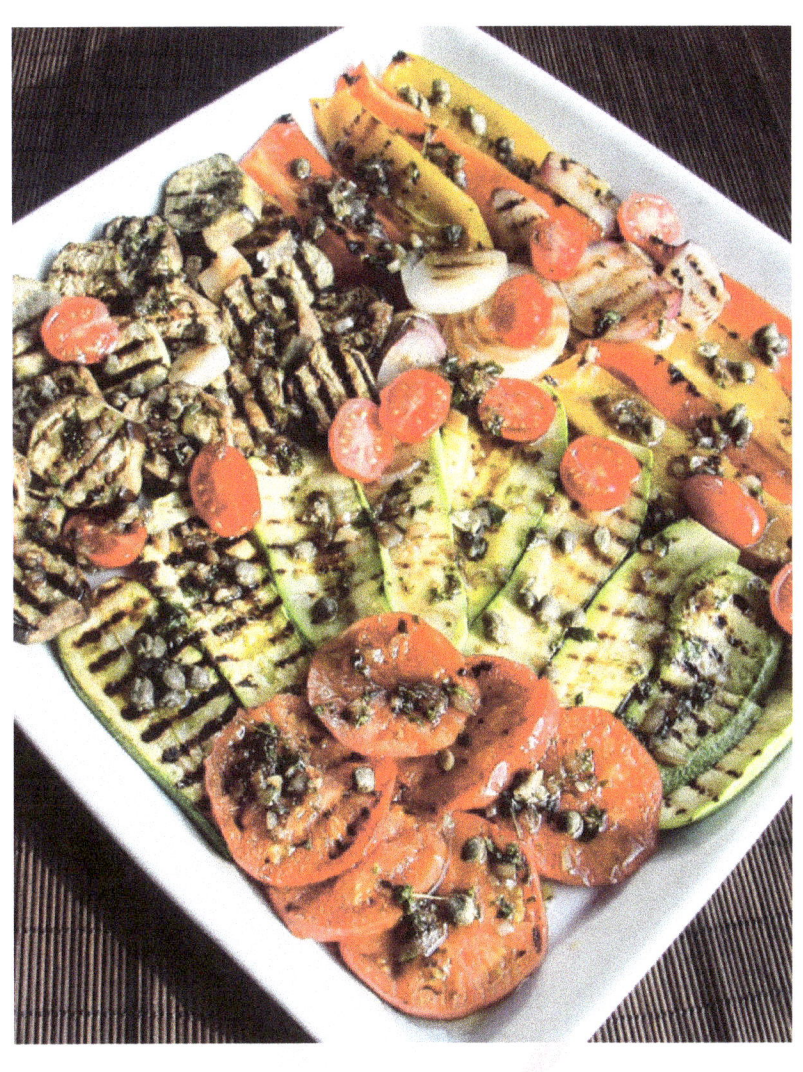

Energizing Breakfast Protein Bars

Total time: 45 minutes
Prep time: 10 minutes
Cook time: 35 minutes
Yield: 6 servings

Ingredients

- ¼ cup pecans, chopped
- 2 tbsp. pistachios, chopped
- ¼ cup flaxseeds, ground
- 1 ¼ cup spelt flakes
- ½ cup dried cherries
- 1 pinch sea salt
- ½ cup honey
- 2 tbsp. extra virgin olive oil
- ¼ cup peanut butter, natural
- ½ tsp. vanilla extract

Directions

- Start by preheating your oven to 325°F, then brush your baking tray with oil.
- Line the baking tray with parchment paper all round and brush it with oil.
- Combine the pecans, pistachios, flaxseeds, spelt, cherries, and salt in a mixing bowl and set aside.
- Place a saucepan over medium heat and pour in the honey, oil, peanut butter, and vanilla extract and cook, stirring, until the mixture melts.

- Add this mixture to the bowl of dry ingredients and mix well.
- Pour the mixture into the prepared baking tray and smooth the top.
- Bake until it turns golden brown and the sides pull out from the edges of the pan.
- Transfer the baked bar from the tray and cut it into smaller sizes on a cutting board.
- After cooling, store in an airtight container lined with parchment paper.
- The bars can last up to one week.

Fruity Nutty Muesli

Total time: 1 hour 15 minutes

Prep time 15 minutes

Cook time 1 hour

Yield: 2 servings

Ingredients

- ⅓ cup almonds, chopped
- ¾ cup oats, toasted
- ½ cup low-fat milk
- ½ cup low-fat Greek yogurt
- ½ green apple, diced
- 2 tbsp. raw honey

Directions

- Preheat oven to 350°F. Place the almonds on a baking sheet and bake until they turn golden brown, about 10 minutes.
- After cooling, mix with the toasted oats, milk and yogurt in a bowl and cover.
- Refrigerate this mixture for an hour until the oats are soft.
- Divide the muesli between two bowls, add the apple and drizzle the honey.

Egg Veggie Scramble

Total time: 30 minutes

Prep time 15 minutes

Cook time 15 minutes

Yield: 2 servings

Ingredients

- 2 tsp. extra virgin olive oil, divided
- 1 medium orange bell pepper, diced
- ½ cup frozen corn kernels
- 1 scallion, thinly sliced
- ¼ tsp. cumin, freshly ground
- ¼ tsp. allspice, plus a pinch
- 2 eggs
- 2 egg whites
- Pinch of cinnamon
- ⅓ cup white cheddar, shredded
- 1 medium avocado, diced
- ½ cup fresh salsa
- 2 whole-wheat flour tortillas, warmed

Directions

- Heat a teaspoon of olive oil in a nonstick pan over medium heat.
- Add bell pepper, tossing and turning for 5 minutes until soft; add the corn, scallion, cumin, and allspice and cook for a further 3 minutes until the scallion wilts.

- Pour this out onto a plate and cover it with foil. Wipe the pan clean with a paper towel and set it aside.
- Place the eggs and egg whites in a bowl and whisk them together with 2 teaspoons of water, a pinch of allspice and a pinch of cinnamon.
- Heat the remaining olive oil in the pan over medium heat and add the egg mixture.
- Cook until the bottom sets, about 30 seconds, then stir gently.
- Continue stirring for about 2 minutes, then add the shredded cheese and vegetables that you had wrapped in foil. Serve with avocado, salsa and the tortillas.

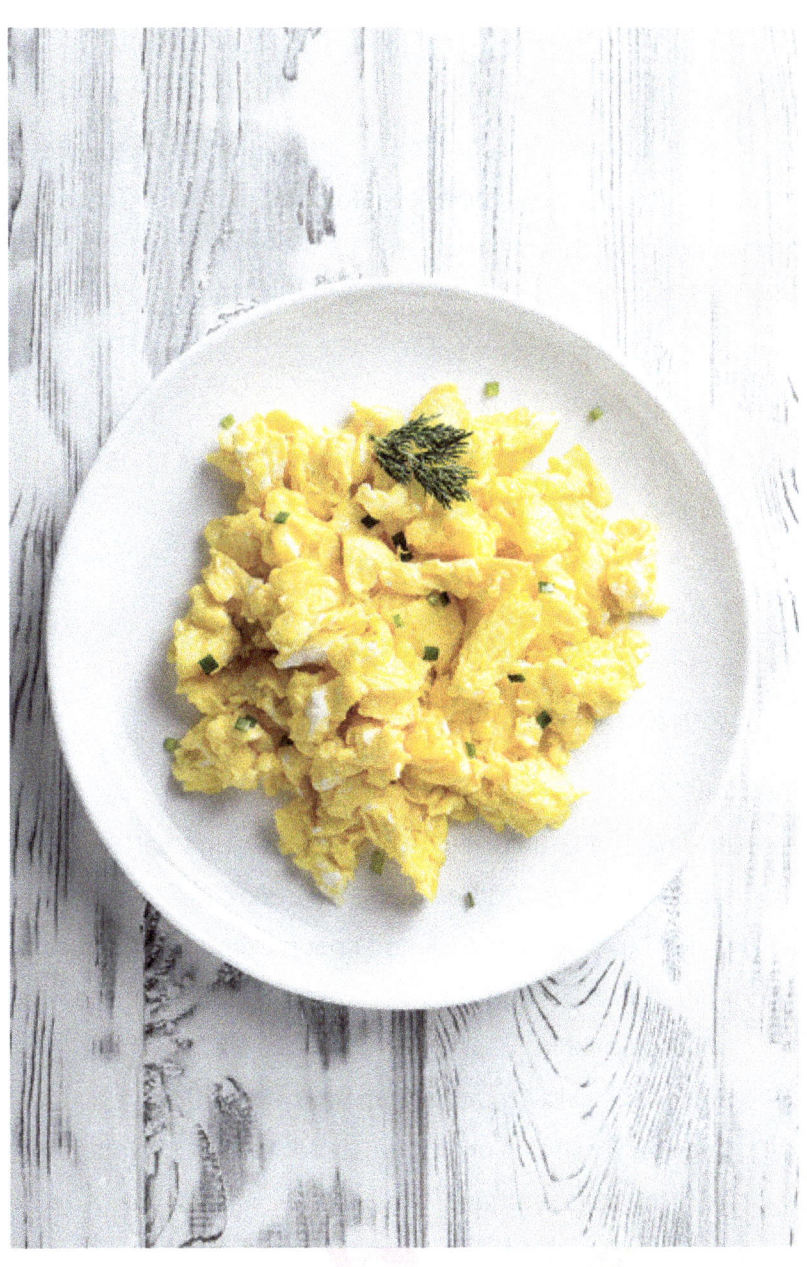

STRAPATSATHA

Strapatsatha is a dish brought to Greece by the Sephardic Jews from Spain. It's a loose omelet of tomatoes and feta. There are many variations of this classic dish.

Serves 4

- 1/4 cup extra-virgin olive oil
- 2/3 cup sliced chorizo sausage
- 4 large ripe tomatoes, passed through a box grater
- 1/2 cup diced sweet banana pepper
- 3 scallions, ends trimmed and sliced
- 1 cup crumbled feta cheese
- 8 large eggs, beaten
- 1/2 teaspoon pepper

Directions

- Add oil to a large skillet over medium-high heat, and heat for 30 seconds. Add sausage and cook for 2 minutes or until it browns. With a slotted spoon, remove the sausage from the skillet and reserve. Take the skillet off the heat and let it cool for 5 minutes.
- Return the skillet to a medium heat and add the tomatoes. Cook for 5 minutes or until most of the water is evaporated. Add the peppers and scallions, and cook for 2 more minutes. Add the feta and cook for 1 minute.
- Add the eggs, pepper, and cooked sausage. Stir the eggs to scramble them, cooking them until they form a loose omelet. Serve immediately or warm.

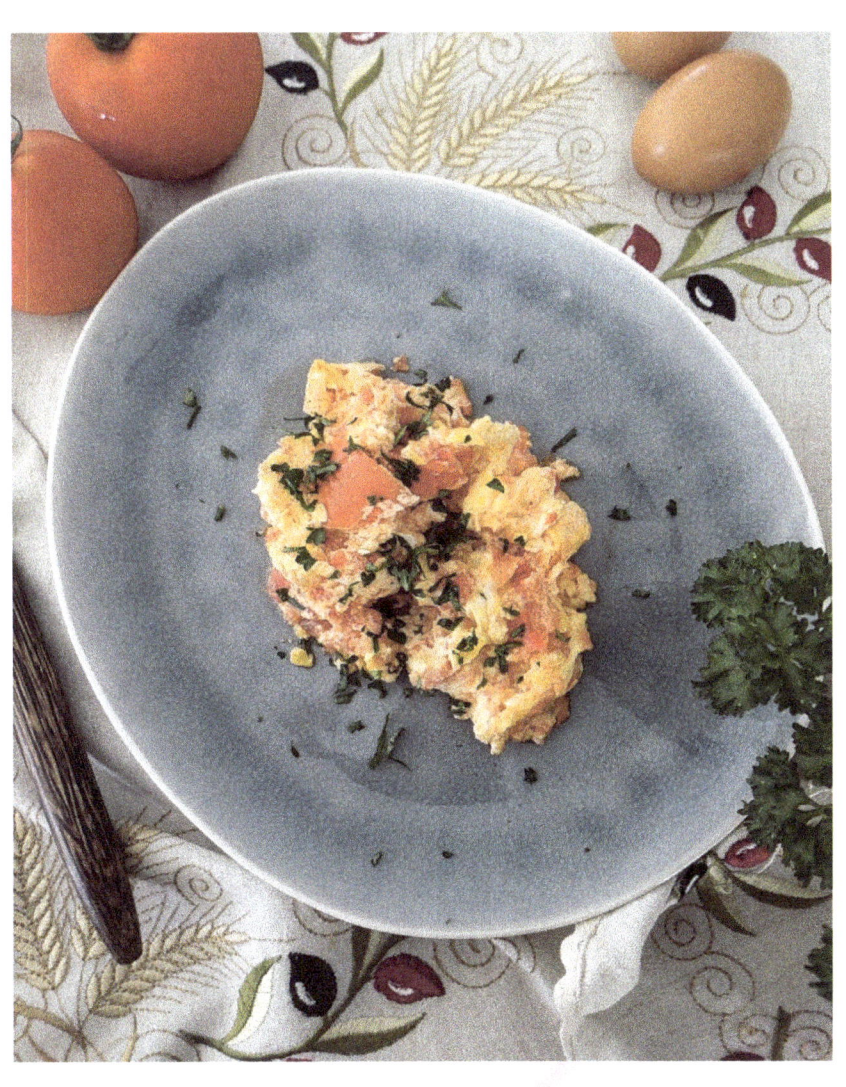

MEDITERRANEAN LUNCH RECIPE

Slow-Cooker Mediterranean Stew

Ingredients

- 2 (14 ounce) cans no-salt-added fire-roasted diced tomatoes
- 3 cups low-sodium vegetable broth
- 1 cup coarsely chopped onion
- ¾ cup chopped carrot
- 4 cloves garlic, minced
- 1 teaspoon dried oregano
- ¾ teaspoon salt
- ½ teaspoon crushed red pepper
- ¼ teaspoon ground pepper
- 1 (15 ounce) can no-salt-added chickpeas, rinsed, divided
- 1 bunch lacinato kale, stemmed and chopped (about 8 cups)
- 1 tablespoon lemon juice
- 3 tablespoons extra-virgin olive oil
- Fresh basil leaves, torn if large
- 6 lemon wedges (Optional)

Directions

- Combine tomatoes, broth, onion, carrot, garlic, oregano, salt, crushed red pepper and pepper in a 4-quart slow cooker. Cover and cook on Low for 6 hours.
- Measure 1/4 cup of the cooking liquid from the slow cooker into a small bowl. Add 2 tablespoons chickpeas; mash with a fork until smooth.

- Add the mashed chickpeas, kale, lemon juice and remaining whole chickpeas to the mixture in the slow cooker. Stir to combine. Cover and cook on Low until the kale is tender, about 30 minutes.
- Ladle the stew evenly into 6 bowls; drizzle with oil. Garnish with basil. Serve with lemon wedges, if desired.

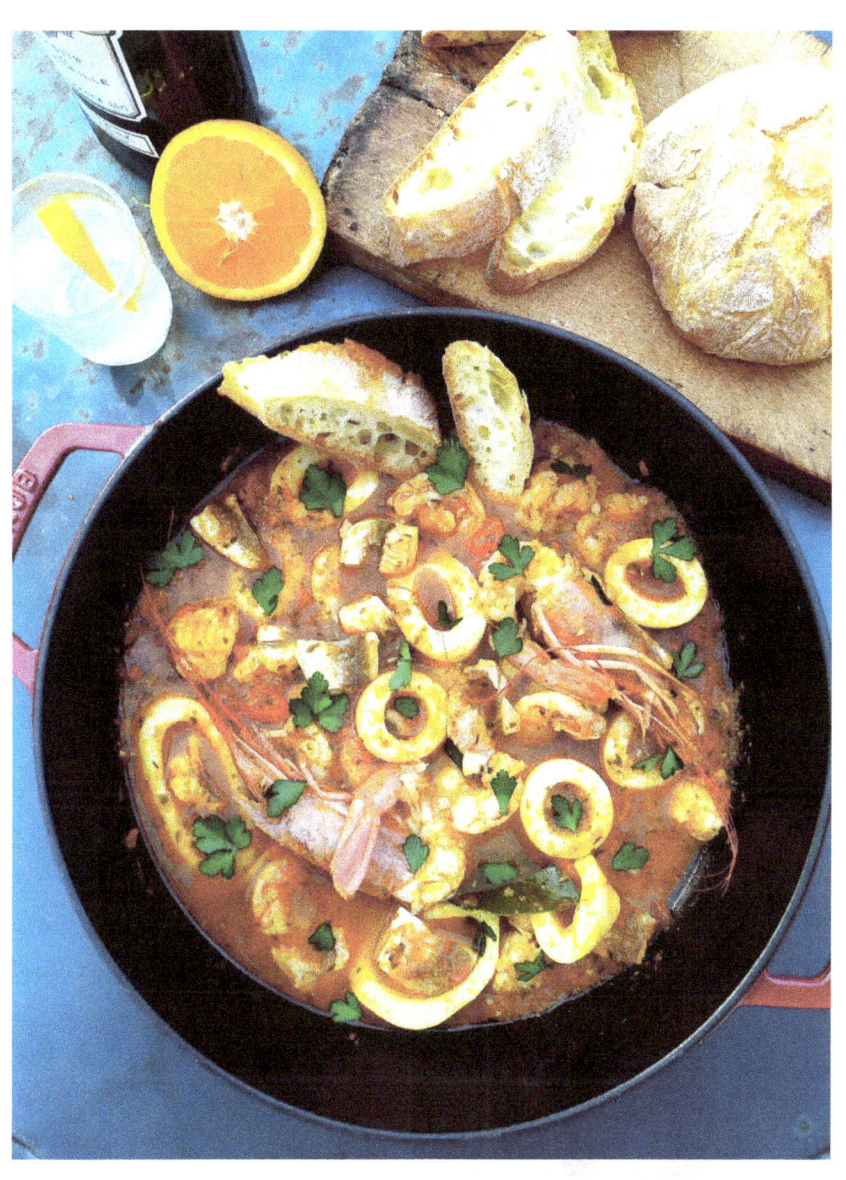

Greek Cauliflower Rice Bowls with Grilled Chicken

Ingredients

- 6 tablespoons plus 1 teaspoon extra-virgin olive oil, divided
- 4 cups cauliflower rice (see Tip)
- ⅓ cup chopped red onion
- ¾ teaspoon salt, divided
- ½ cup chopped fresh dill, divided
- 1 pound boneless, skinless chicken breasts
- ½ teaspoon ground pepper, divided
- 3 tablespoons lemon juice
- 1 teaspoon dried oregano
- 1 cup halved cherry tomatoes
- 1 cup chopped cucumber
- 2 tablespoons chopped Kalamata olives
- 2 tablespoons crumbled feta cheese
- 4 wedges Lemon wedges for serving

Directions

- Preheat grill to medium.
- Heat 2 tablespoons oil in a large skillet over medium-high heat. Add cauliflower, onion and 1/4 teaspoon salt. Cook, stirring occasionally, until the cauliflower is softened, about 5 minutes. Remove from heat and stir in 1/4 cup dill.
- Meanwhile, rub 1 teaspoon oil all over chicken. Sprinkle with 1/4 teaspoon salt and 1/4 teaspoon pepper. Grill,

turning once, until an instant-read thermometer inserted into the thickest part of the breast reads 165 degrees F, about 15 minutes total. Slice crosswise.

- Meanwhile, whisk the remaining 4 tablespoons oil, lemon juice, oregano and the remaining 1/4 teaspoon each salt and pepper in a small bowl.
- Divide the cauliflower rice between 4 bowls. Top with the chicken, tomatoes, cucumber, olives and feta. Sprinkle with remaining 1/4 cup dill. Drizzle with the vinaigrette. Serve with lemon wedges, if desired.

Prosciutto Pizza with Corn & Arugula

Ingredients

- 1 pound pizza dough, preferably whole-wheat
- 2 tablespoons extra-virgin olive oil, divided
- 1 clove garlic, minced
- 1 cup part-skim shredded mozzarella cheese
- 1 cup fresh corn kernels
- 1 ounce very thinly sliced prosciutto, torn into 1-inch pieces
- 1 ½ cups arugula
- ½ cup torn fresh basil
- ¼ teaspoon ground pepper

Directions

- Preheat grill to medium-high. (Or to bake instead, see Tips.)
- Roll dough out on a lightly floured surface into a 12-inch oval. Transfer to a lightly floured large baking sheet. Combine 1 tablespoon oil and garlic in a small bowl. Bring the dough, the garlic oil, cheese, corn and prosciutto to the grill.
- Oil the grill rack (see Tips). Transfer the crust to the grill. Grill the dough until puffed and lightly browned, 1 to 2 minutes.
- Flip the crust over and spread the garlic oil on it. Top with the cheese, corn and prosciutto. Grill, covered, until the cheese is melted and the crust is lightly browned on the

bottom, 2 to 3 minutes more. Return the pizza to the baking sheet.
- Top the pizza with arugula, basil and pepper. Drizzle with the remaining 1 tablespoon oil.

Cheesy Spinach-&-Artichoke Stuffed Spaghetti Squash

Ingredients

- 1 (2 1/2 to 3 pound) spaghetti squash, cut in half lengthwise and seeds removed
- 3 tablespoons water, divided
- 1 (5 ounce) package baby spinach
- 1 (10 ounce) package frozen artichoke hearts, thawed and chopped
- 4 ounces reduced-fat cream cheese, cubed and softened
- ½ cup grated Parmesan cheese, divided
- ¼ teaspoon salt
- ¼ teaspoon ground pepper
- Crushed red pepper & chopped fresh basil for garnish

Directions

- Place squash cut-side down in a microwave-safe dish; add 2 tablespoons water. Microwave, uncovered, on High until tender, 10 to 15 minutes. (Alternatively, place squash halves cut-side down on a rimmed baking sheet. Bake at 400 degrees F until tender, 40 to 50 minutes.)
- Meanwhile, combine spinach and the remaining 1 tablespoon water in a large skillet over medium heat. Cook, stirring occasionally, until wilted, 3 to 5 minutes. Drain and transfer to a large bowl.
- Position rack in upper third of oven; preheat broiler.

- Use a fork to scrape the squash from the shells into the bowl. Place the shells on a baking sheet. Stir artichoke hearts, cream cheese, 1/4 cup Parmesan, salt and pepper into the squash mixture. Divide it between the squash shells and top with the remaining 1/4 cup Parmesan. Broil until the cheese is golden brown, about 3 minutes. Sprinkle with crushed red pepper and basil, if desired.

Vegan Mediterranean Lentil Soup

Ingredients

- 2 tablespoons extra-virgin olive oil
- 1 ½ cups chopped yellow onions
- 1 cup chopped carrots
- 3 cloves garlic, minced
- 2 tablespoons no-salt-added tomato paste
- 4 cups reduced-sodium vegetable broth
- 1 cup water
- 1 (15 ounce) can no-salt-added cannellini beans, rinsed
- 1 cup mixed dry lentils (brown, green and black)
- ½ cup chopped sun-dried tomatoes in oil, drained
- ¾ teaspoon salt
- ½ teaspoon ground pepper
- 1 tablespoon chopped fresh dill, plus more for garnish
- 1 ½ teaspoons red-wine vinegar

Directions

- Heat oil in a large heavy pot over medium heat. Add onions and carrots; cook, stirring occasionally, until softened, 3 to 4 minutes. Add garlic and cook, stirring constantly, until fragrant, about 1 minute. Add tomato paste and cook, stirring constantly, until the mixture is evenly coated, about 1 minute.
- Stir in broth, water, cannellini beans, lentils, sun-dried tomatoes, salt and pepper. Bring to a boil over medium-high heat; reduce heat to medium-low to maintain a

simmer. Cover and simmer until the lentils are tender, 30 to 40 minutes.
- Remove from heat and stir in dill and vinegar. Garnish with additional dill, if desired and serve.

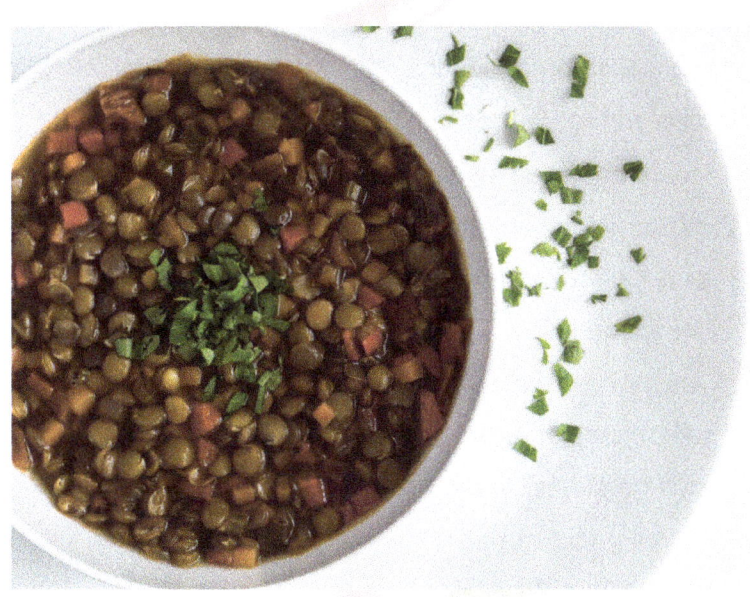

EatingWell's Eggplant Parmesan

Ingredients

- Canola or olive oil cooking spray
- 2 large eggs
- 2 tablespoons water
- 1 cup panko breadcrumbs
- ¾ cup grated Parmesan cheese, divided
- 1 teaspoon Italian seasoning
- 2 medium eggplants (about 2 pounds total), cut crosswise into ¼-inch-thick slices
- ½ teaspoon salt
- ½ teaspoon ground pepper
- 1 (24 ounce) jar no-salt-added tomato sauce
- ¼ cup fresh basil leaves, torn, plus more for serving
- 2 cloves garlic, grated
- ½ teaspoon crushed red pepper
- 1 cup shredded part-skim mozzarella cheese, divided

Directions

- Position racks in middle and lower thirds of oven; preheat to 400°F. Coat 2 baking sheets and a 9-by-13-inch baking dish with cooking spray.
- Whisk eggs and water in a shallow bowl. Mix breadcrumbs, 1/4 cup Parmesan and Italian seasoning in another shallow dish. Dip eggplant in the egg mixture, then coat with the breadcrumb mixture, gently pressing to adhere.

- Arrange the eggplant in a single layer on the prepared baking sheets. Generously spray both sides of the eggplant with cooking spray. Bake, flipping the eggplant and switching the pans between racks halfway, until the eggplant is tender and lightly browned, about 30 minutes. Season with salt and pepper.
- Meanwhile, mix tomato sauce, basil, garlic and crushed red pepper in a medium bowl.
- Spread about 1/2 cup of the sauce in the prepared baking dish. Arrange half the eggplant slices over the sauce. Spoon 1 cup sauce over the eggplant and sprinkle with 1/4 cup Parmesan and 1/2 cup mozzarella. Top with the remaining eggplant, sauce and cheese.
- Bake until the sauce is bubbling and the top is golden, 20 to 30 minutes. Let cool for 5 minutes. Sprinkle with more basil before serving, if desired.

BBQ Shrimp with Garlicky Kale & Parmesan-Herb Couscous

Ingredients

- 1 cup low-sodium chicken broth
- ¼ teaspoon poultry seasoning
- ⅔ cup whole-wheat couscous
- ⅓ cup grated Parmesan cheese
- 1 tablespoon butter
- 3 tablespoons extra-virgin olive oil, divided
- 8 cups chopped kale
- ¼ cup water
- 1 large clove garlic, smashed
- ¼ teaspoon crushed red pepper
- ¼ teaspoon salt
- 1 pound peeled and deveined raw shrimp (26-30 per pound)
- ¼ cup barbecue sauce (see Tip)

Directions

- Combine broth and poultry seasoning in a medium saucepan over medium-high heat. Bring to a boil. Stir in couscous. Remove from heat, cover and let stand for 5 minutes. Fluff with a fork, then stir in Parmesan and butter. Cover to keep warm.
- Meanwhile, heat 1 tablespoon oil in large skillet over medium-high heat. Add kale and cook, stirring, until bright green, 1 to 2 minutes. Add water, cover and cook, stirring

occasionally, until the kale is tender, about 3 minutes. Reduce heat to medium-low. Make a well in the center of the kale and add 1 tablespoon oil, garlic and crushed red pepper; cook, undisturbed, for 15 seconds, then stir the garlic oil into the kale and season with salt. Transfer to a bowl and cover to keep warm.
- Add the remaining 1 tablespoon oil and shrimp to the pan. Cook, stirring, until the shrimp are pink and curled, about 2 minutes. Remove from heat and stir in barbecue sauce. Serve the shrimp with the kale and couscous.

MEDITERRANEAN SALAD RECIPES

LAHANOSALATA (CABBAGE SALAD)

Serves 4

- 1/3 of a white cabbage
- 2 large carrots
- 1/2 cup Greek-style strained yogurt
- 1/4 cup extra-virgin olive oil
- 2 tablespoons fresh lemon juice (or vinegar)
- 1/2 teaspoon dried oregano
- 1 tablespoon chopped fresh dill Salt and pepper to taste

Directions

- Wash cabbage well; peel carrots. Shred cabbage finely with a sharp knife. Shred carrots into ribbons using a mandoline or the large holes on a grater; add to shredded cabbage.
- Toss shredded cabbage and carrots well.
- In a food processor/blender, add yogurt, olive oil, lemon juice, oregano, dill, salt, and pepper; blend together until smooth and creamy.
- Pour the dressing over the top of individual servings or mix well into the entire salad before serving. Garnish with chopped dill and a kalamata olive or two.

TARAMOSALATA/TARAMA (FISH ROE SALAD)

Serves 6–8

- ½ loaf two-day-old white bread
- ½ cup carp roe 1 large onion, grated Juice of 2 lemons
- 2 cups extra-virgin olive oil
- Cucumber slices, for garnish
- Tomato slices, for garnish
- Olives, for garnish

Directions

- Remove the outside crust and soak the inner bread in water; squeeze well to drain and set aside.
- Place fish roe in a food processor/blender; mix a minute or so to break down eggs.
- Add grated onion to the processor; continue mixing.
- Add moistened bread in stages to the processor/blender; mix well.
- Slowly add lemon juice and olive oil while constantly mixing. Note: When adding olive oil and lemon juice, add in a slow and alternate fashion by first adding some lemon juice then some olive oil and so on, until both are incorporated into the tarama.
- Refrigerate before serving to firm up the tarama. Garnish with cucumber, tomato slices, and/or olive(s); serve with warm pita bread.

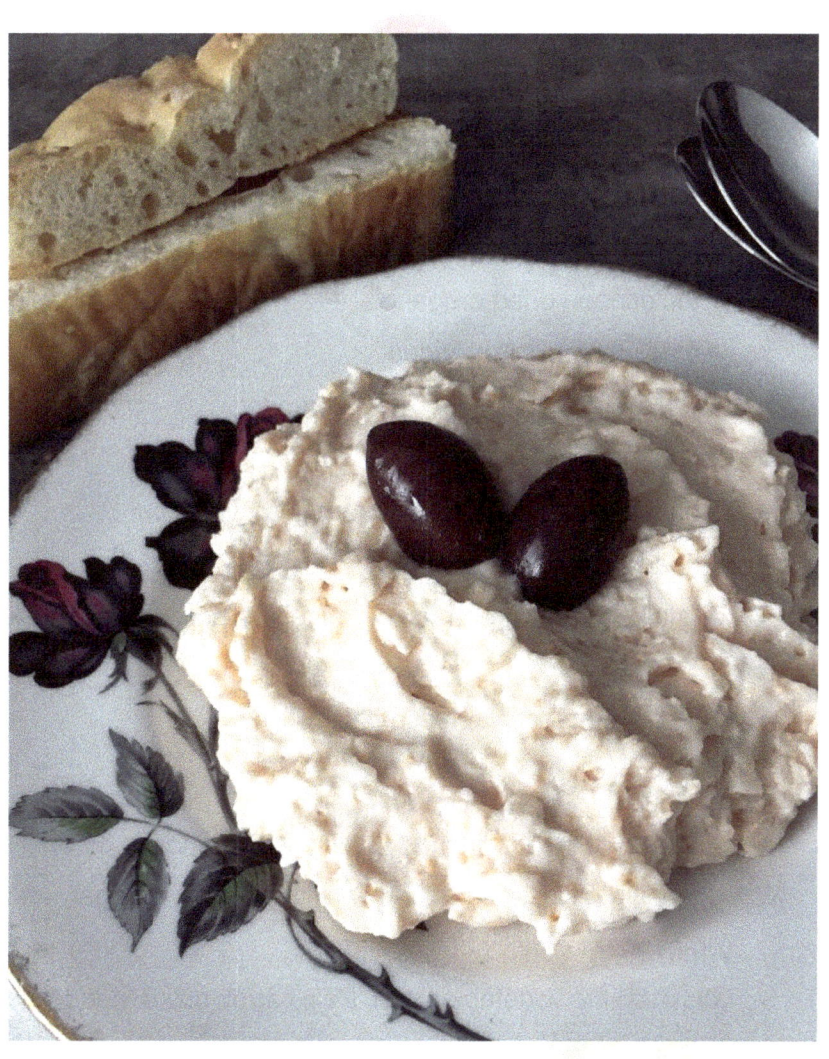

GRILLED HALLOUMI SALAD

Serves 4

- 10–12 kalamata olives, pitted and finely chopped or ground to a pulp
- 1/4 cup extra-virgin olive oil 2 tablespoons balsamic vinegar
- 1 tablespoon dried oregano
- 1 medium carrot, shredded
- 1/4 of a small green cabbage, shredded
- 1 large tomato
- 1 bunch fresh rocket greens (arugula), finely cut
- 1 head romaine lettuce, finely cut
- 2 stalks fresh green onion, finely sliced (green stalk included)
- 1/2 pound halloumi cheese, thick sliced

Directions

- Prepare the dressing by pitting and grinding or finely chopping olives; combine pulp with olive oil, vinegar, and oregano. Mix well; set aside.
- Wash all the vegetables well. Peel carrot; use a mandoline to finely shred cabbage and carrot into a large salad bowl. Chop tomato into sections; add to the bowl. Finely cut rocket and lettuce; add to the bowl. Finely slice green onions; add to salad.
- Fire up a grill; grill the halloumi until it noticeably starts to soften and grill marks appear. Make sure to flip the cheese

so both sides are scored with grill marks. When the cheese is done, remove from heat and immediately cut into cubes; add to salad. Pour dressing over the salad; mix well. Serve immediately.

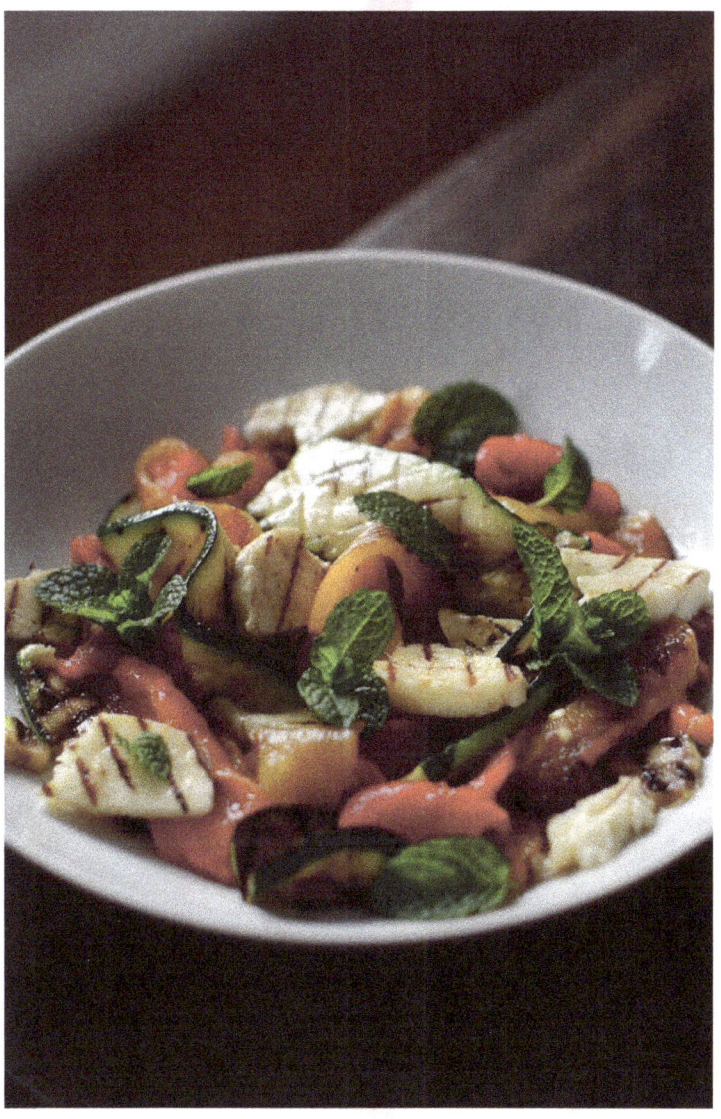

MEDITERRANEAN POULTRY RECIPES

CHICKEN GALANTINE

Serves 6

- 1 small whole chicken
- 1 shallot
- 2 cloves garlic
- 1/4 cup pistachio nuts 8 dates
- 1/2 pound ground chicken 1 egg white
- 1 teaspoon dried oregano
- 1 teaspoon dried marjoram
- Fresh-cracked black pepper, to taste
- Kosher salt, to taste

Directions

- Preheat the oven to 325°F.
- Carefully remove all the skin from the chicken by making a slit down the back and loosening the skin with your fingers (keep the skin intact as much as possible); set aside the chicken and the skin. Remove the breast from bone. Chop the shallot and mince the garlic. Chop the nuts and dates.
- Mix together the ground chicken, egg white, nuts, dates, shallots, garlic, oregano, marjoram, pepper, and salt.
- Lay out the skin, then lay the breast lengthwise at the center. Spoon the ground chicken mixture on top, and fold over the rest of skin. Place in a loaf pan and bake for 1 1/2–2 hours (when the internal temperature of the loaf reaches 170° F, it's done). Let cool, then slice.

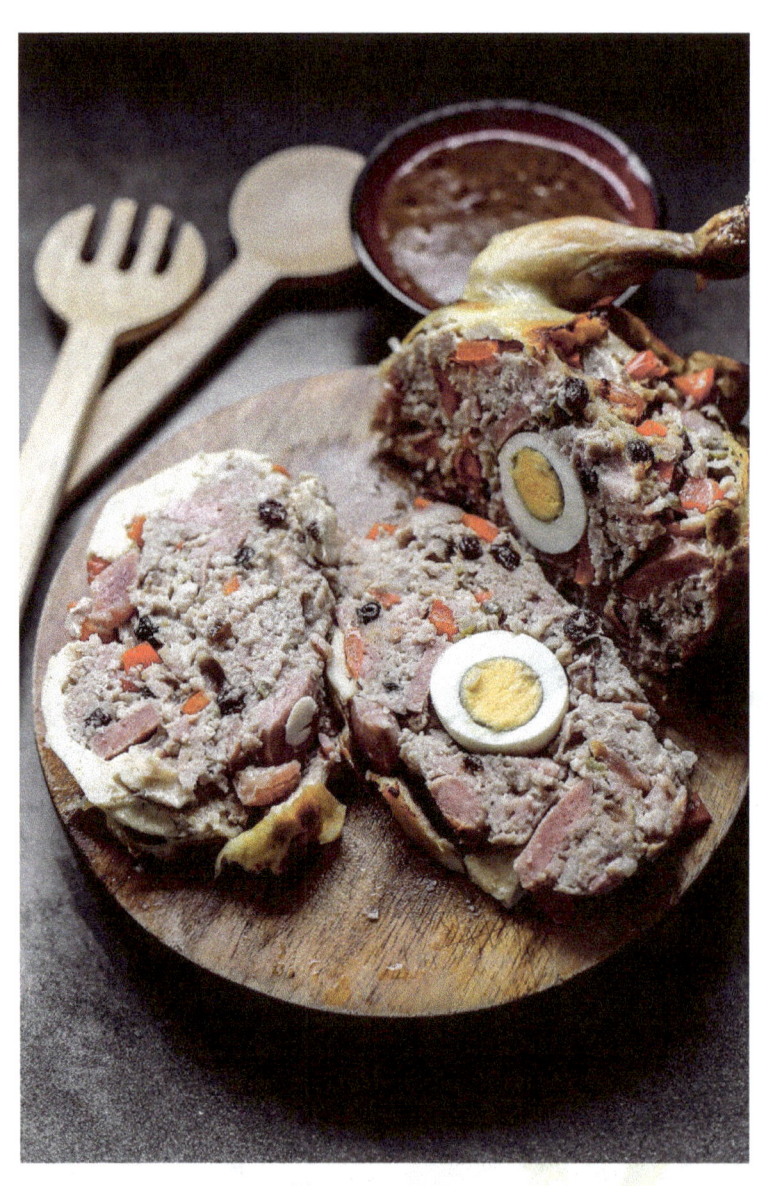

SPICY TURKEY BREAST WITH FRUIT CHUTNEY

Serves 6

- 2 jalapeño chili peppers
- 2 cloves garlic
- 1 tablespoon olive oil
- 2 teaspoons all-purpose flour
- Fresh-cracked black pepper, to taste
- Cooking spray
- 1½ pounds whole boneless turkey breast 1 shallot
- lemon
- 2 pears
- tablespoon honey
- 1 pomegranate

Directions

- Preheat the oven to 350°F.
- Stem, seed, and mince the peppers. Mince the garlic. In a blender, purée the chili peppers, garlic, and oil. Mix together the flour and black pepper.
- Spray a rack with cooking spray. Dredge the turkey in the flour mixture, then dip it in the pepper mixture, and place on rack. Cover loosely with foil and roast for 1 hour. Remove foil and brown for 10 minutes.
- While the turkey cooks, prepare the chutney: Finely dice the shallots. Juice the lemon and grate the rind for zest.

Dice the pears. Mix together the pears, shallot, lemon juice, zest, and honey.
- Thinly slice the turkey, and serve with chutney.

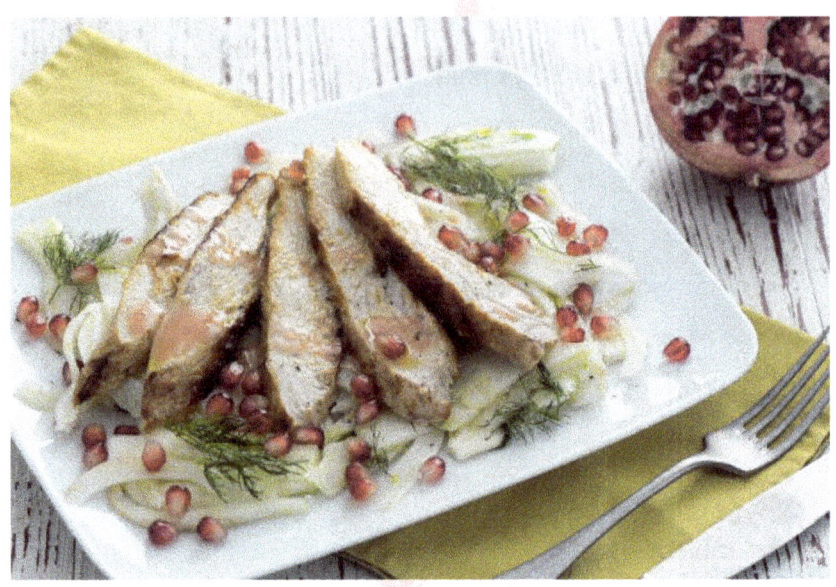

GRILLED DUCK BREAST WITH FRUIT SALSA

Serves 6

- plum
- peach
- nectarine
- red onion
- 3 sprigs mint
- Fresh-cracked black pepper, to taste
- tablespoon olive oil
- teaspoon chili powder
- 1 1/2 pounds boneless duck breast

Directions

- Preheat the grill. Dice the plum, peach, nectarine, and onion. Mince the mint. Toss together the fruit, onion, mint, and pepper.
- Mix together the oil and chili powder. Dip the duck breast in the oil, and cook to desired doneness on grill.
- Slice duck on the bias and serve with a spoonful of salsa.

QUAIL WITH PLUM SAUCE

Serves 6

- quail 12 plums
- 2 yellow onions
- 1 stalk celery
- 1 carrot
- 1/4 cup olive oil 2 bay leaves
- 1 cup dry red wine
- 1 quart Hearty Red Wine Brown Stock
- 2 sprigs thyme, leaves only
- 1/2 bunch parsley stems Kosher salt, to taste Fresh-cracked black pepper, to taste

Directions

- Cut the quail in half and remove breast and back bones (reserve bones). Peel, pit, and chop the plums. Chop the onions and celery. Peel and chop the carrot.
- Heat the oil to medium-high temperature in a large stockpot. Brown the quail bones, then add the onions, carrots, and celery, and brown slightly. Add the plums and wine, and let reduce by half.
- Add the stock and herbs; simmer for 6 hours, then strain, removing bay leaves.
- Preheat grill.
- Season the quail meat with the salt and pepper; grill on each side until golden brown. Serve with stock.

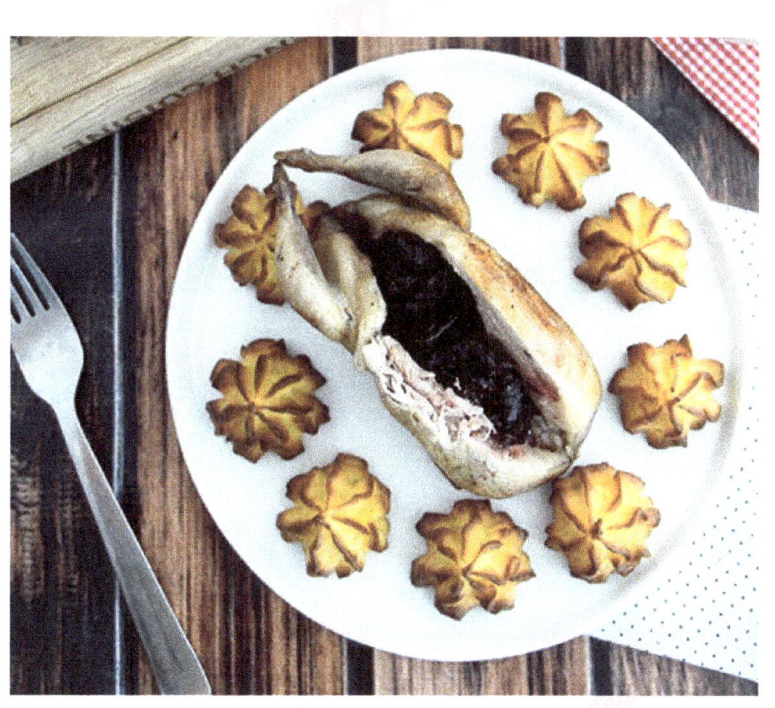

MEDITERRANEAN SEAFOOD RECIPES

STEAMED SEAFOOD DINNER

Serves 6

- 1 pound lobster
- 1/2 dozen clams 1/2 dozen oysters
- 1/2 dozen mussels
- 1/2 dozen large shrimp 1/2 dozen sea scallops 3 large potatoes
- 1/2 dozen carrots 1/2 bunch fresh parsley
- 1/2 dozen celery stalks 6 shallots
- 6 small sprigs thyme
- 1/2 cup white wine (Pinot Grigio or Sauvignon Blanc) Juice of 1 lemon
- 1 cup Seafood Stock
- 3 bay leaves
- 1/2 teaspoon Old Bay Seasoning Fresh-cracked black pepper, to taste

Directions

- Clean the shellfish thoroughly in ice-cold water. Cut the potatoes in half. Peel the carrots (leave whole). Chop the parsley. (Leave the celery and shallots whole.)
- In a medium-size saucepot, bring the wine, lemon juice, and stock to a boil. Add the potatoes, carrots, celery, shallots, herbs, and spices; let simmer for 45 minutes. Add the rest of the ingredients and reduce to a simmer; cook for 10–15 more minutes. Remove the thyme sprigs, then serve.

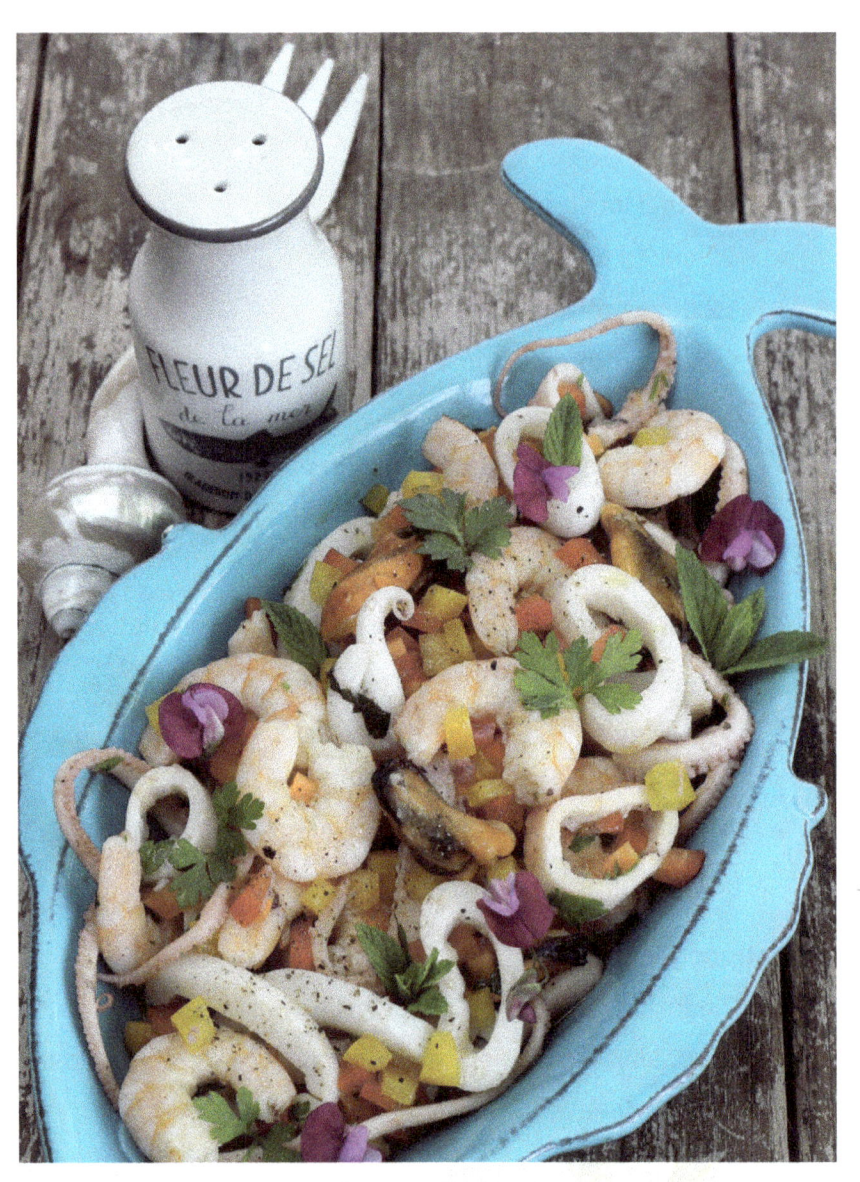

GRILLED FISH WITH POLENTA

Serves 6

- 1/2 serrano chili pepper 2 teaspoons olive oil
- 1 quart Fish Stock
- 1 1/2 cups cornmeal 1 teaspoon extra-virgin olive oil
- 1 1/2 pounds red snapper Pinch of coarse sea salt Fresh-cracked black pepper, to taste
- 3 ounces manchego cheese
- 1 tablespoon cider vinegar

Directions

- Preheat grill to medium heat. Stem, seed, and dice the serrano chili pepper.
- Heat the olive oil in a stockpot over medium heat. Lightly sauté the chili, then add the stock and bring to a boil.
- Whisk in the cornmeal slowly; cook for approximately 20–30 minutes, stirring frequently (add more broth if necessary).
- While the polenta cooks, lightly dip the fish in the extra-virgin olive oil and place on a rack to drain. Season with salt and pepper.
- When the polenta is done cooking, remove it from the heat and add the manchego; keep warm.
- Grill the fish for 3–5 minutes on each side, depending on the thickness of the fish.

- To serve, spoon out a generous dollop of polenta on each serving plate and arrange the fish on top. Drizzle with the vinegar.

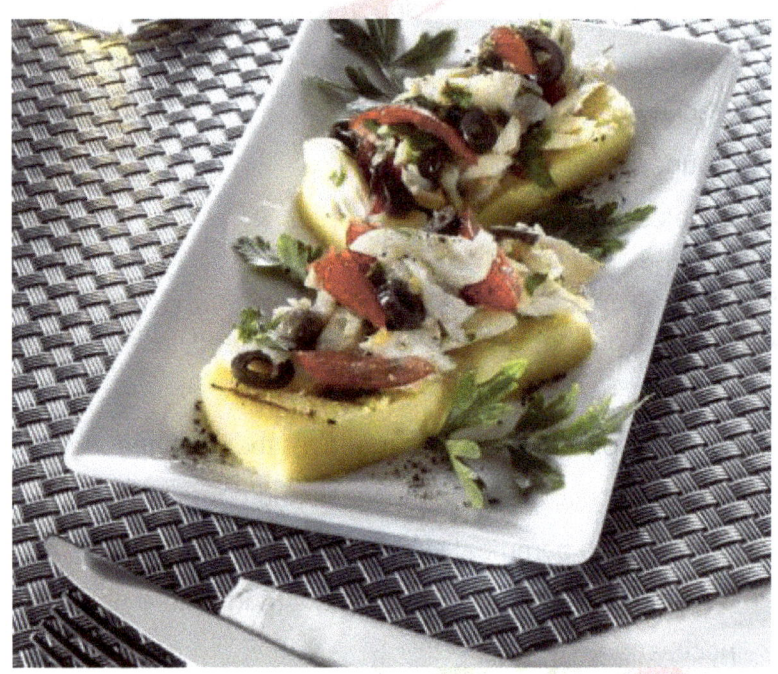

BACCALÁ

Serves 6

- 1 1/2 pounds baccalá (salted cod) 3 cloves garlic
- 2 plum tomatoes
- 1 stalk celery
- 1/2 bunch fresh parsley
- 1 tablespoon olive oil
- 1/4 cup dry white wine
- 1/2 cup Fish Stock
- Fresh-cracked black pepper, to taste

Directions

- Soak the baccalá for 24 hours in water.
- Mince the garlic. Medium-dice the tomatoes and celery. Mince the parsley.
- Heat the oil in a large sauté pan over medium-high heat. Add the baccalá, garlic, tomatoes, and celery; sauté the baccalá on each side for approximately 1 minute. Add the wine and let it reduce by half. Add the stock and pepper; simmer, covered, for 10 minutes.
- Serve with the cooking liquid and sprinkle with parsley.

FLOUNDER WITH BALSAMIC REDUCTION

Serves 6

- 1/4 cup all-purpose flour 1 tablespoon cornmeal
- 1 1/2 pounds flounder 1 tablespoon olive oil
- 1/2 cup Balsamic Reduction
- Fresh-cracked black pepper, to taste
- 3 sprigs dill

Directions

- Mix together the flour and cornmeal; coat the flounder in the mixture.
- Heat the oil over medium heat in a large sauté pan. Cook the flounder for approximately 7 minutes on each side.
- While the flounder cooks, heat the Balsamic Reduction sauce. Serve the fish drizzled with the sauce and sprinkled with pepper; garnish each serving with half a sprig of dill.

MEDITERRANEAN MEAT, BEEF AND PORK RECIPES

AUBERGINE MEAT ROLLS

Serves 4–6

- 1 large, round eggplant
- 1 large white onion, finely diced
- 1/2 cup Greek extra-virgin olive oil, divided 2 cloves garlic, minced or pressed
- 1 pound lean ground veal
- 1/2 cup white wine (or Retsina)
- 2 cups strained tomato pulp/juice
- 1 teaspoon ground cumin
- Salt and pepper to taste
- Flour for dredging
- 1 cup shredded or grated Greek Graviera cheese (or mild Gruyère)
- 1/3 cup dried bread crumbs 2 tablespoons finely chopped fresh mint
- 1/3 cup pine nuts 1 egg

Directions

- Preheat the oven to 350°F.
- Wash eggplant thoroughly and remove stalk. Slice thinly along its length; aim for 12 slices. Salt both sides and spread in a flower pattern in a colander. Set aside to drain for 30 minutes. Remember to flip the slices at least once for better drainage.
- In a large frying pan over medium-high heat, sauté onions in 1/4 cup olive oil until soft; stir garlic in for 1 minute. Add

- meat and mix well; sauté for 8–10 minutes to brown it thoroughly. Set aside while you prepare tomato sauce.
- Add wine, 2 cups tomato juice, cumin, salt, and pepper to a small pot; stir well to mix completely. Bring to a boil and simmer over medium-low heat for 30 minutes, stirring occasionally. Once sauce has completely reduced, remove frying pan from heat and set aside to cool.
- Heat 3 tablespoons olive oil in a large fry pan. Lightly flour both sides of the eggplant slices; fry in batches until softened. Add olive oil to pan as needed, but do it in a thin stream around the entire circumference of the pan so it seeps toward the center. Shake the frying pan back and forth with each batch to keep eggplant slices from sticking to the bottom. Once the eggplant slices have been lightly fried, spread on paper towels in a pan.
- Retrieve the cooled meat mixture. In a large mixing bowl, add cheese (leave aside a few tablespoonfuls of shredded cheese for use as a garnish later), bread crumbs, mint, pine nuts, and egg; mix well to combine with meat. Pick up an eggplant slice; place a heaping spoonful of meat mixture in the middle of one end. Roll up that end to complete a full end-to-end overlapping roll; use a toothpick to pin in place. Be sure not to press the center of the roll too hard, as you do not want the meat to protrude from the open sides.
- Place rolls side by side in close rows in a deep-walled pan greased with olive oil. Spoon tomato sauce on top of rolls

in single stripe right along the middle of the rolled slices; sprinkle cheese on top of the tomato sauce stripe.
- Bake for 30 minutes. Let stand to cool for at least 10 minutes before serving. Garnish with a little more shredded cheese while still warm.

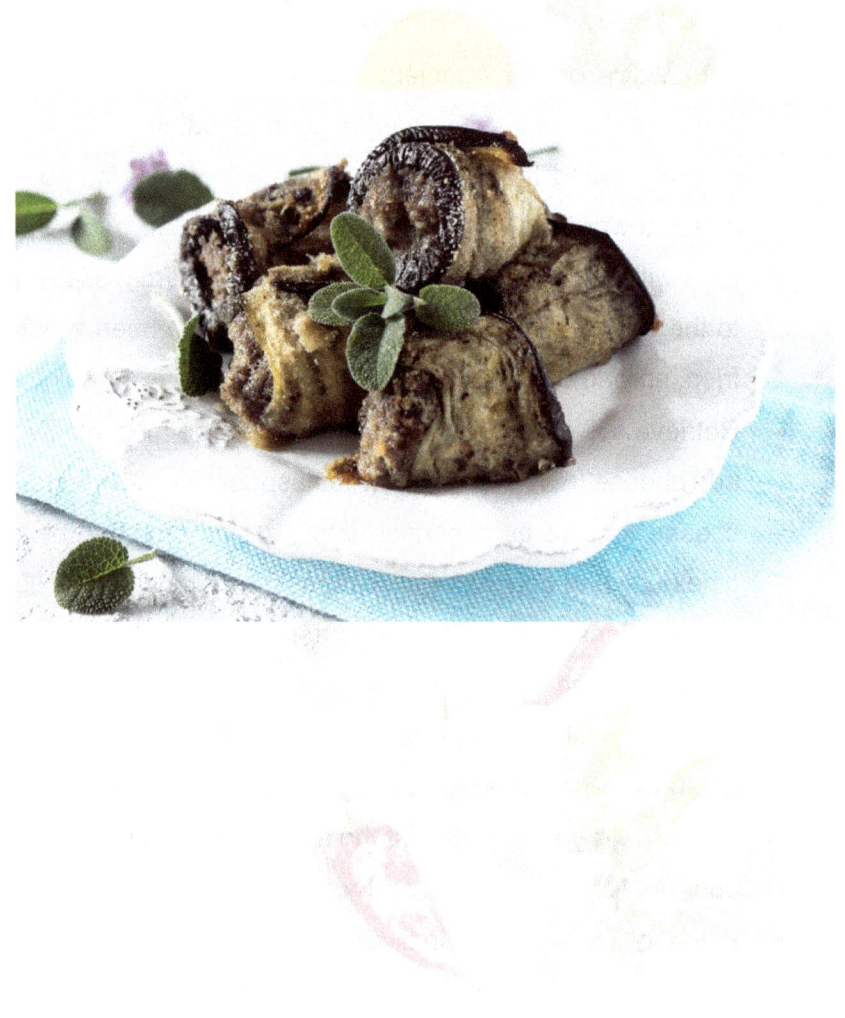

PORK WITH LEEKS AND CELERY

Serves 4

- 2 pounds pork shoulder, chopped into cubes
- 1 onion, finely chopped
- 1/2 cup extra-virgin olive oil 1/2 cup white wine 2 cups water
- 2 pounds leeks
- 1 cup finely chopped celery
- 1 cup tomatoes, diced and sieved (fresh or canned)
- 1 teaspoon dried oregano
- Salt and fresh-ground pepper

Directions

- Wash pork well; chop into cubes and set aside to drain.
- In a deep-walled pot, sauté onion in olive oil until slightly soft; add pork and brown thoroughly.
- Add wine to the pot; bring to a boil, then cover and simmer for 15 minutes, stirring regularly. Remove pork; cover to keep warm and set aside.
- Add water to the pan along with the leeks and celery; bring to a boil and simmer for 30 minutes over medium heat.
- Return pork to the pot along with tomatoes, oregano, salt, and pepper; stir well. Bring to a boil and continue to simmer until the sauce is reduced and thickened, approximately 8–10 minutes. Serve immediately.

STIFADO (BRAISED BEEF WITH ONIONS)

Serves 4

- 1/2 cup extra-virgin olive oil 2 pounds stewing beef, cubed
- 2 tablespoons tomato paste, diluted in 2 cups of water
- 2 tablespoons wine vinegar (or a sweet dessert wine like Madeira or Mavrodaphne)
- 16 pearl onions, peeled
- 6 cloves garlic, peeled
- 4 spice cloves
- 1 small cinnamon stick
- 1 tablespoon dried oregano
- Salt and fresh-ground pepper

Directions

- Add olive oil to a large pot over medium-high heat; add meat and brown well on all sides by stirring continuously so meat does not stick to the bottom of the pot.
- Add tomato paste, wine vinegar, onions, garlic, cloves, cinnamon, oregano, salt, and pepper; mix well and turn heat to high. Bring to a boil.
- Cover and turn heat down to medium-low; simmer for approximately 1 hour.
- Serve immediately, accompanied by fresh bread for sauce.

BRAISED LAMB SHOULDER

Serves 4

- 1 1/2–2 pounds lamb shoulder
- 1/2 cup extra-virgin olive oil
- 1/2 cup hot water
- 2 cups tomatoes, diced and sieved (fresh or canned)
- 2 bay leaves
- 4 cloves garlic, peeled and minced
- 1 cinnamon stick
- 1 tablespoon dried thyme
- Salt and pepper to taste

Directions

- Wash meat well and cut into small pieces; include bones.
- Heat olive oil in a pot; brown meat on all sides.
- Add water, tomatoes, bay leaves, garlic, cinnamon, thyme, salt, and pepper; cover and bring to a boil, then turn heat down to medium-low.
- Simmer for 1 1/2 hours, stirring occasionally.

VEGETARIAN AND LEGUMES MEDITERRANEAN RECIPES

KIDNEY BEAN CASSEROLE

Serves 6

- 1 teaspoon olive oil
- 1/4 bunch celery
- 1 yellow onion
- 1/2 head romaine lettuce
- 1 cup puréed carrots
- 1 cup Basic Vegetable Stock
- 1 cup cooked kidney beans
- 1/2 cup cooked barley 3 sprigs thyme, leaves only
- 1/2 teaspoon dried oregano leaves
- 1/2 teaspoon chili powder Fresh-cracked black pepper, to taste

Directions

- Preheat the oven to 325°F. Grease a casserole or loaf pan with the oil.
- Slice the celery and onion. Shred the romaine lettuce.
- Blend together the carrot purée and stock.
- In the prepared dish, layer the beans, celery, onions, barley, herbs, spices, and the carrot-stock mixture; cover and bake for 30–45 minutes. Serve topped with shredded romaine.

LENTIL AND WALNUT CHILI

Serves 6

- 2 cups red lentils
- 1/2 cup walnuts 2 shallots
- 4 cloves garlic
- 2 poblano peppers
- 1 tablespoon olive oil
- 1 1/2 cups Basic Vegetable Stock
- 2 1/2 cups Fresh Tomato Sauce
- 1 teaspoon cumin
- 1 1/2 tablespoons chili powder 1 tablespoon honey
- 1/2 cup plain nonfat yogurt (optional)

Directions

- Lay out the lentils on a baking sheet and pick out any stones. Chop the walnuts and slice the shallots. Mince the garlic and dice the peppers.
- Heat the oil over medium heat in a saucepot. Add the shallots, garlic, and peppers; sauté for 1–2 minutes. Add all the remaining ingredients except the lentils and yogurt. Simmer for 1 hour, then add the lentils and cook for 30 minutes longer.
- Ladle into bowls. Serve with a dollop of yogurt.

RED LENTIL LASAGNA

Serves 6

- 1 tablespoon olive oil
- 2 cups Béchamel Sauce
- 1 pound cooked lasagna noodles
- 1/2 cup crumbled firm tofu
- 1/2 cup cooked red lentils
- 1/4 cup peeled and shredded carrots
- 1 yellow onion, chopped
- 4 cloves garlic, minced
- 1/2 cup cooked chopped spinach
- 1 sprig fresh oregano, chopped
- 1 sprig fresh marjoram, chopped
- Fresh-cracked black pepper, to taste

Directions

- Preheat the oven to 325°F.
- Brush a casserole dish with the olive oil. Alternate all the ingredients in the dish in layers, starting with a thin layer of sauce to moisten the bottom before the first layer of noodles, and ending with the Béchamel Sauce on top. Cover tightly and bake for 30–45 minutes. Cool slightly, cut, and serve.

GRILLED PORTOBELLO MUSHROOMS

Serves 6

- 6 portobello mushrooms
- 3 cloves garlic
- 1 tablespoon olive oil
- Kosher or coarse sea salt, to taste
- Fresh-cracked black pepper, to taste

Directions

- Preheat the grill to medium temperature. Clean off the mushrooms with damp paper towels or a mushroom brush, and scrape out the black membrane on the underside of the cap. Mince the garlic.
- Mix together the oil and garlic; dip each mushroom in the oil and place on a rack to drain. Season with salt and pepper, and grill on each side until fork-tender.
- To serve, slice on the bias and fan out on serving plates.

MEDITERRANEAN DESSERTS

FRESH FRUIT AND MERINGUE

Serves 12

- 6 egg whites
- 1/2 cup granulated sugar
- 1/4 teaspoon cream of tartar 2 cups chopped fresh fruit
- 1/4 teaspoon fresh-grated lemon zest 1/2 pound chopped almonds 3 tablespoons honey
- Preheat the oven to 200°F.

Directions

- Line a baking sheet with parchment paper or spray with cooking spray.
- In a copper or stainless steel bowl, beat the egg whites, sugar, and cream of tartar until stiff. Drop by the spoonful on baking sheet and bake in the oven for 5–6 hours, until dry, crispy, and lightly golden.
- Serve with fresh seasonal fruit. Sprinkle with lemon zest, almonds, and honey.

POACHED APPLES

Serves 6

- 6 Granny Smith apples
- lemon
- cup apple cider
- 1/4 cup sweet white wine 3 whole cloves or 1/4 teaspoon ground cloves 2 cinnamon sticks or 1/2 teaspoon ground cinnamon 1/4 cup golden raisins or confectionery sugar

Directions

- Peel the apples (coring optional). Zest and juice the lemon.
- Place the apples in a large saucepan with the cider, wine, lemon juice, zest, cloves, and cinnamon; simmer, covered, on medium heat for 30–45 minutes, until the apples are fork tender. Remove apples and keep warm.
- Reduce the cooking liquid. Serve apples sprinkled with raisins.

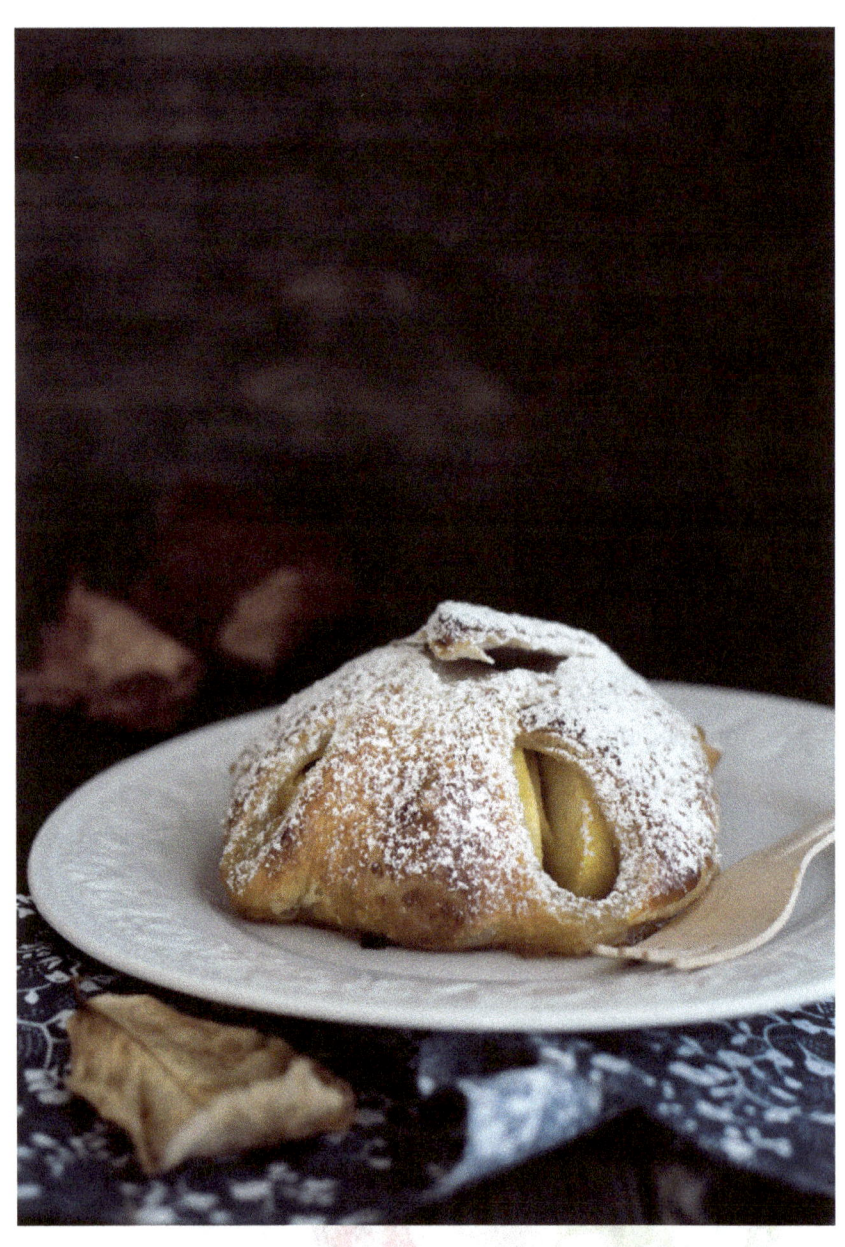

CINNAMON ALMOND CAKE

Serves 12

- 1 cup sugar
- 1/4 teaspoon grated lemon rind 6 egg yolks
- 1/2 pound finely ground almonds
- 1/2 teaspoon cinnamon 6 egg whites
- 1/2 cup heavy cream
- 1/4 teaspoon granulated sugar
- 1 teaspoon brandy
- Chopped almonds, for garnish

Directions

- Preheat oven to 350°F.
- Cream the sugar, rind, and yolks until light and fluffy. Stir in finely ground almonds and cinnamon.
- Whip the egg whites until stiff. Stir a few tablespoons of whites into the almond mixture and then fold in the rest.
- Pour into 2 greased 8-inch pans; bake for 45 minutes. Let cool briefly and remove from pans.
- Whip the cream with the sugar and brandy. Spread between cake layers and then on top and sides. Garnish with chopped almonds.

Decorated Figs

Total time: 1 hour 10 minutes

Prep time: 15 minutes

Cook time: 40 minutes

Cooling time: 15 minutes

Yield: 6 servings

Ingredients

- 1 cup dry red wine
- ½ cup sugar
- ½ cup balsamic vinegar
- 1 pound dried figs, remove stems
- ½ cup mascarpone
- ¾ cup toasted and chopped walnuts

Directions

- Preheat oven to 350°F and place oven rack in mid position.
- Pour the wine, sugar and vinegar in a nonstick saucepan and bring to a boil over medium heat, stirring constantly until the sugar dissolves.
- Add figs to the pan and simmer for 5 minutes.
- Pour the contents of the saucepan into a ceramic baking dish and top with walnuts.
- Bake in preheated oven for about 30 minutes until the figs absorb most of the liquid.
- Set aside and let it cool for about 15 minutes then serve with the sauce and a generous topping of mascarpone.

MEDITERRANEAN BREAD

PASTOURMA PIE

Serves 12

- 1 package phyllo pastry, thawed and at room temperature
- 1 cup butter, melted
- 16 thin slices pastourma
- 3 medium tomatoes, thinly sliced
- 1½ cups Béchamel Sauce
- ½ pound sliced kasseri or Havarti cheese

Directions

- Divide the phyllo sheets into two equal piles, take two sheets from one pile, and add them to the other pile. The pile with a greater number of sheets will form the bottom layer, and the other pile will form the top layer. Cover each pile with a slightly damp tea towel so the phyllo doesn't dry out. Brush the bottom and sides of a 13" × 9" rectangular or square pan with the butter.
- Take one sheet of phyllo from the bottom layer pile, and brush the surface with the butter. Place the sheet in the bottom of the pan with a quarter of the sheet hanging over the side of the pan. Continue buttering and laying the bottom-layer sheets in the pan until the entire bottom and edges are covered with phyllo.
- Add a layer of pastourma over the bottom layer of phyllo. Then add a layer of tomatoes. Spread the Béchamel Sauce over the tomatoes. Top with a layer of cheese.

- Take one sheet from the top-layer pile and brush the surface with butter. Place the sheet on top of the filling (butter side up) and repeat with the remaining sheets to cover the entire surface of the pan. If excess phyllo is hanging from the edges of the pan, gently tuck the excess into the sides of the pan. Chill the pie for 30 minutes.
- Preheat the oven to 350°F. With a sharp knife, score the top layers of phyllo into serving squares, about 1/4-inch deep.
- Bake the pie on the middle rack for 45 minutes or until the pie is golden. Let the pie cool for 15–20 minutes before serving.

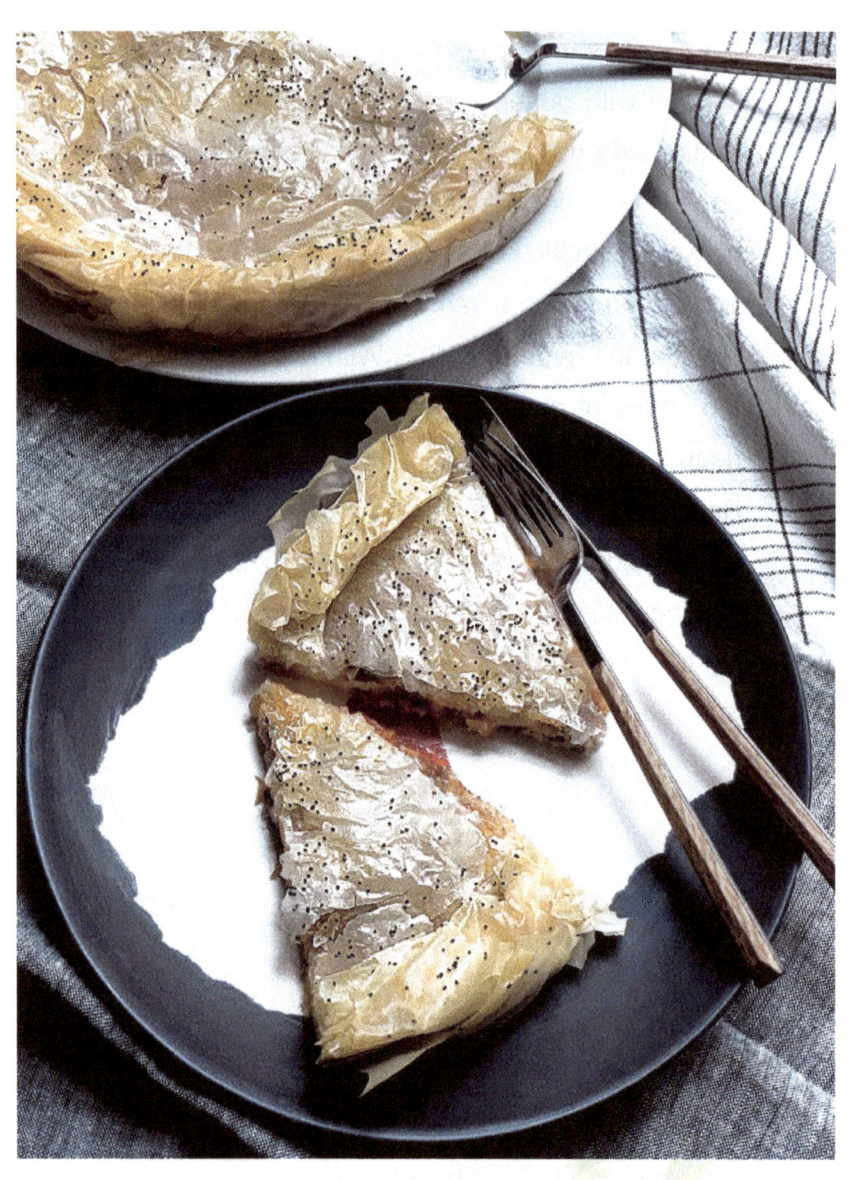

PRASSOPITA (LEEK PIE)

Serves 6

- 1/2 cup extra-virgin olive oil
- 3 or 4 large leeks, sliced thinly (upper dark-green stalks removed)
- 1/4 cup green onion, finely chopped
- 3 large eggs
- 1 1/2 cups milk 1 cup crumbled Greek feta cheese
- 3/4 cup all-purpose flour
- 1/4 cup fresh dill, finely chopped
- 1 teaspoon dried oregano
- Fresh-ground pepper and pinch of salt

Directions

- Preheat the oven to 350°F.
- Heat olive oil in pan; sauté leeks about 5 minutes. Add onion; continue sautéing until both are soft and tender, another 3 minutes or so.
- In a large bowl, beat eggs well; add milk, feta, flour, dill, oregano, pepper, salt, and sautéed leeks and onions; mix well.
- Grease sides of a baking dish with olive oil; pour mixture into the dish. Bake about 1 hour.
- Allow to cool before cutting. Can be served warm or at room temperature.

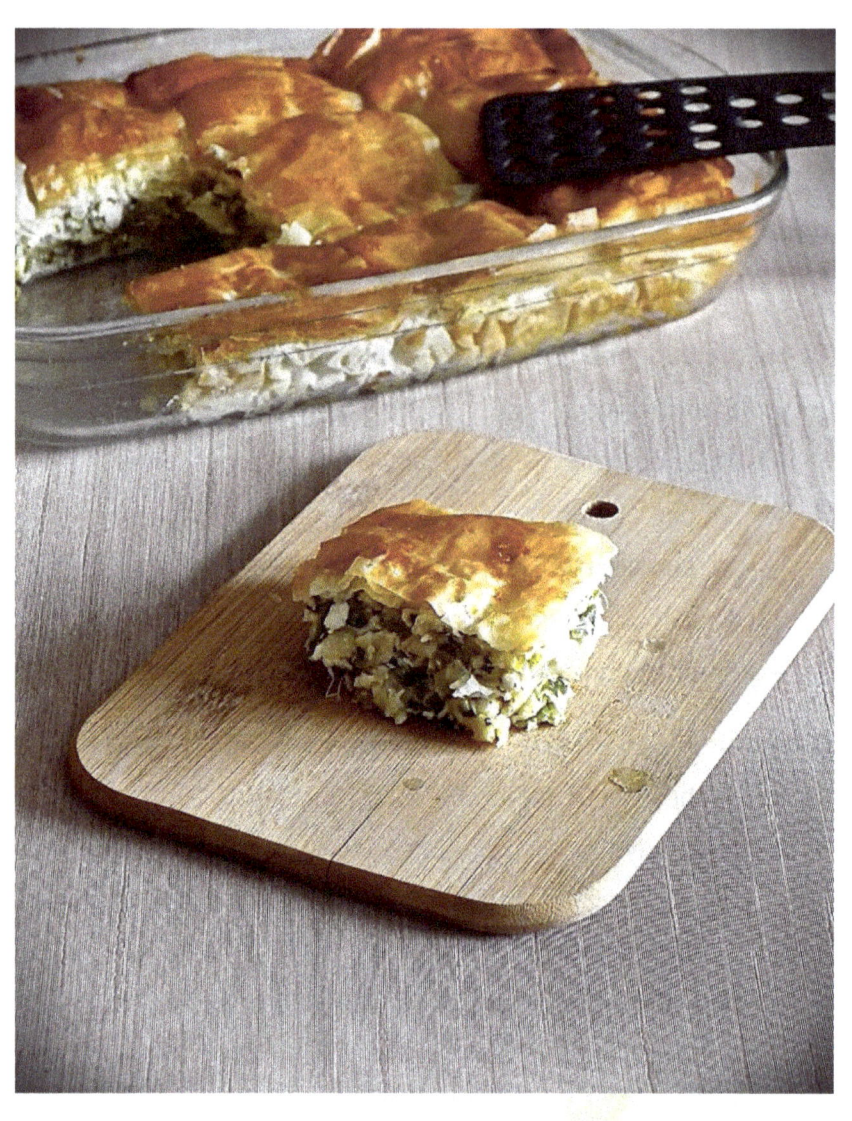

MEDITERRANEAN RICE AND GRAINS

Low Sodium Garlic Parmesan Popcorn

Ingredients

- 2 teaspoons olive or avocado oil
- 1/4 cup popcorn kernels
- 2 cloves garlic, minced
- 2 tablespoons good quality parmesan cheese, freshly grated
- 1/4 teaspoon garlic powder

Preparation

- Heat oil in the bottom of a small saucepan over medium high heat. Add 2 or 3 kernels to the pan while heating.
- Once kernels start to pop, add remaining popcorn kernels and garlic. Cover the pan and cook, shaking the pan to keep kernels from burning.
- Once kernels have stopped popping, remove from heat and sprinkle the parmesan and garlic powder on top. Shake to coat popcorn evenly, then pour into bowls and enjoy.

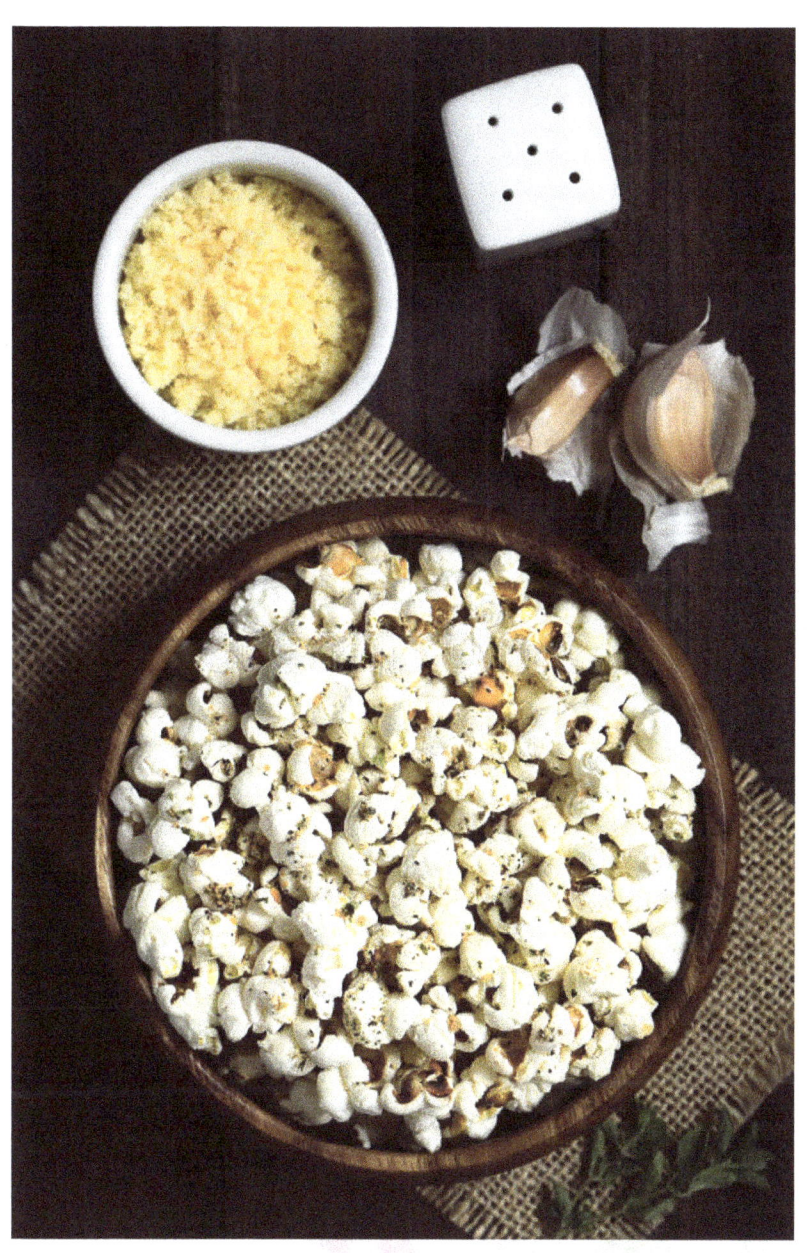

MEDITERRANEAN EGG AND RECIPIES

Mediterranean Egg Mug

Ingredients:
- One farm fresh egg
- 1 Tbsp Trader Joe's Fat Free crumbled Feta cheese (if you don't like Feta sub the Laughing Cow Light Swiss wedge like in my other recipes)
- Diced Mushrooms (I prefer baby bellas)
- Banana pepper rings
- 3 large olives (I try to use Kalamata but black or green work well too)
- Fresh kale and/or baby spinach
- Fresh ground black pepper
- Olive oil non stick spray

Directions
- Spray mug, muffin cooker or crock bowl with non stick spray. Add everything but the egg and cook in microwave on high for 30 seconds
- Crack open egg and add to bowl stirring gently but evenly into the other ingredients.
- Return to microwave for 2 minutes on high. If you have a low wattage microwave or the mixture is still "loose" continue to microwave in 20 second increments until everything is firm but not hard. Add fresh black pepper. Let sit for one minute before trying to remove from bowl to move to bread or plate. The egg "muffin" should slide out

easily. Use your imagination, these are a delicious and quick filling breakfast…enjoy!

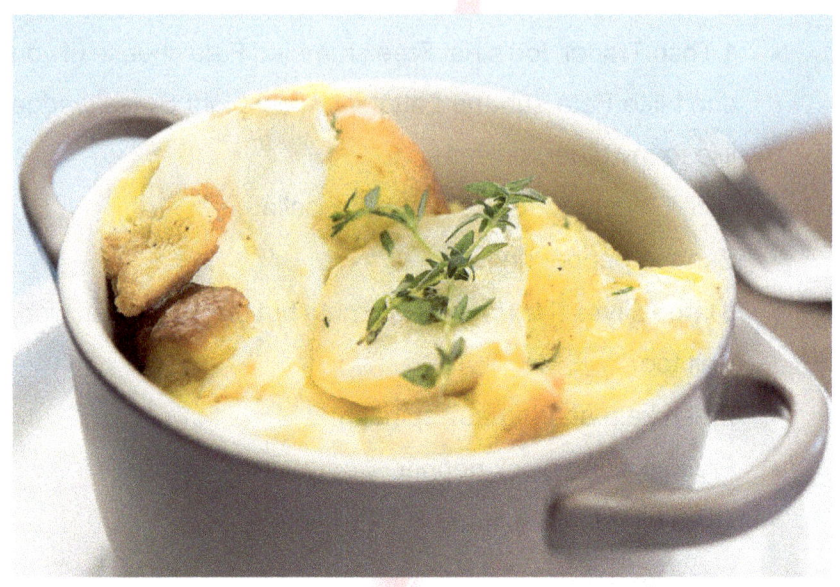

MEDITERRANEAN BREAKFAST BAKE

Texas Traditional Okra Bread

Dry Ingredients

1 cup raw, shell-free sunflower seeds 2¼ cups golden flaxseed meal

1 teaspoon baking soda

1 teaspoon baking powder

2 tablespoons KAL nutritional yeast or your favorite imitation butter powder alternative

1 teaspoon sea salt

Wet Ingredients

- 3 cups chopped fresh okra (about 8 ounces)
- 1 cup chopped tomato
- ½ cup liquid egg whites
- 1 tablespoon vinegar
- 3 whole okra pods, sliced lengthwise into 4 or 5 slivers each

Directions

1. Preheat the oven to 350°F.
2. Cover a 12 × 17-inch baking sheet with Pan Lining Paper, foil side down.
3. Grind sunflower seeds into a fine meal.
4. In a large bowl, mix together dry ingredients.
5. Blend wet ingredients (except sliced okra) thoroughly in blender.
6. Transfer the wet mixture to the bowl of dry ingredients. Mix well and quickly.

7. Scrape the batter onto the prepared baking sheet. Push the mixture to the edges, then level with a spatula. Top with okra slices and bake for about 60 minutes or until dry to the touch.
8. Place upside down on a cooling rack. Remove the pan and paper. Let cool.
9. After cooling, cut into desired pieces or use as a prebaked pizza crust. Store in a sealed container in the refrigerator.

Gratitude Herb Bread

Dry Ingredients

- 1 cup raw, shell-free sunflower seeds
- 3 cups golden flaxseed meal
- ½ teaspoon fresh or dried sage
- 1 teaspoon fresh or dried thyme
- 2 tablespoons onion powder
- 1 teaspoon baking soda
- 2 teaspoons baking powder
- 1 teaspoon sea salt

Wet Ingredients

- 1¼ cups cooked Great Northern beans, or 1 (15.8-ounce) can, drained and rinsed
- 1 cup chopped celery
- 1 cup chopped zucchini
- 4 large eggs
- 2 tablespoons vinegar

Directions

1. Preheat the oven to 350°F.
2. Cover a 12 × 17-inch baking sheet with Pan Lining Paper, foil side down.
3. Grind sunflower seeds into a fine meal.
4. In a large bowl, mix together the dry ingredients.
5. Blend wet ingredients thoroughly in blender.
6. Transfer the wet mixture to the bowl of dry ingredients. Mix well and quickly.

7. Scrape the batter onto the prepared baking sheet. Push the mixture to the edges, then level with a spatula. Bake for about 45 minutes or until dry to the touch.
8. Place upside down on a cooling rack. Remove the pan and paper. Let cool.
9. After cooling, cut into desired pieces or use as a prebaked pizza crust. Store in a sealed container in the refrigerator.

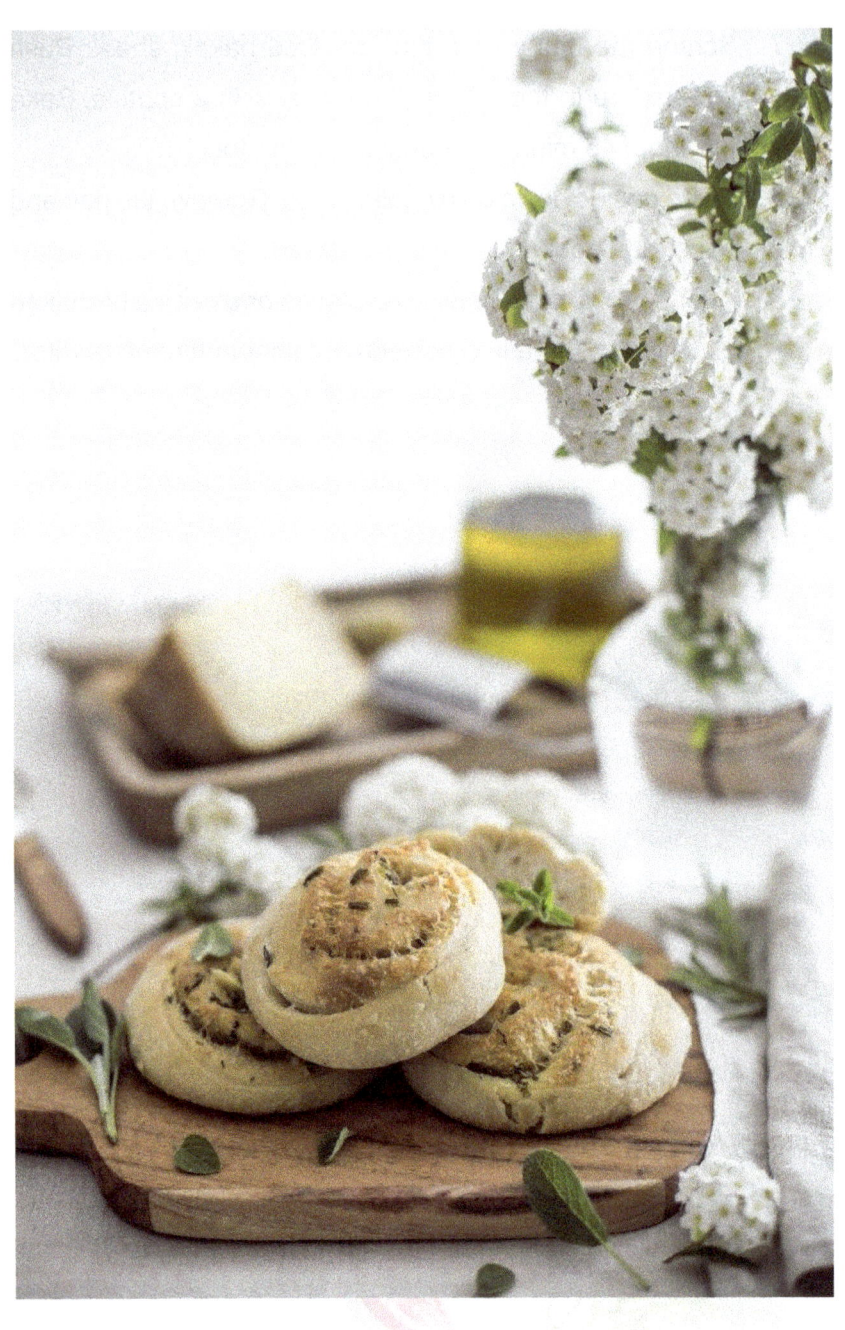

Asian Kale Bread

Dry Ingredients

- 1 cup raw, shell-free pumpkin seeds
- 1½ cups flaxseed meal
- 1 teaspoon each, organic lemongrass and ginger teas (about 1 teabag each)
- 1 teaspoon dehydrated or powdered garlic
- 2 tablespoons whole sesame seeds (optional)
- 1 teaspoon baking soda
- 1½ teaspoons baking powder
- 1 teaspoon sea salt

Wet Ingredients

- 3 medium eggs
- 1 cup chopped red bell pepper
- 1 tablespoon vinegar
- 11 cups fresh baby kale leaves or chopped curly kale (5–6 ounces)
- 2 cups chopped fresh stir-fry vegetables (broccoli, carrots, snow peas)

Directions

1. Preheat the oven to 350°F.
2. Cover a 12 × 17-inch baking sheet with Pan Lining Paper, foil side down.
3. Grind pumpkin seeds into a fine meal.
4. In a large bowl, mix together the dry ingredients.

5. In a blender, combine wet ingredients in order listed. Blend very well, completely breaking up the fresh vegetables into the liquid.
6. Transfer the vegetable mixture to the bowl of dry ingredients. Mix quickly and well.
7. Scrape the batter onto the prepared baking sheet. Push the mixture to the edges, then level with a spatula. Bake for about 50 minutes or until dry to the touch.
8. Place upside down on a cooling rack. Remove the pan and paper. Let cool.
9. After cooling, cut into desired pieces or use as a prebaked pizza crust. Store in a sealed container in the refrigerator.

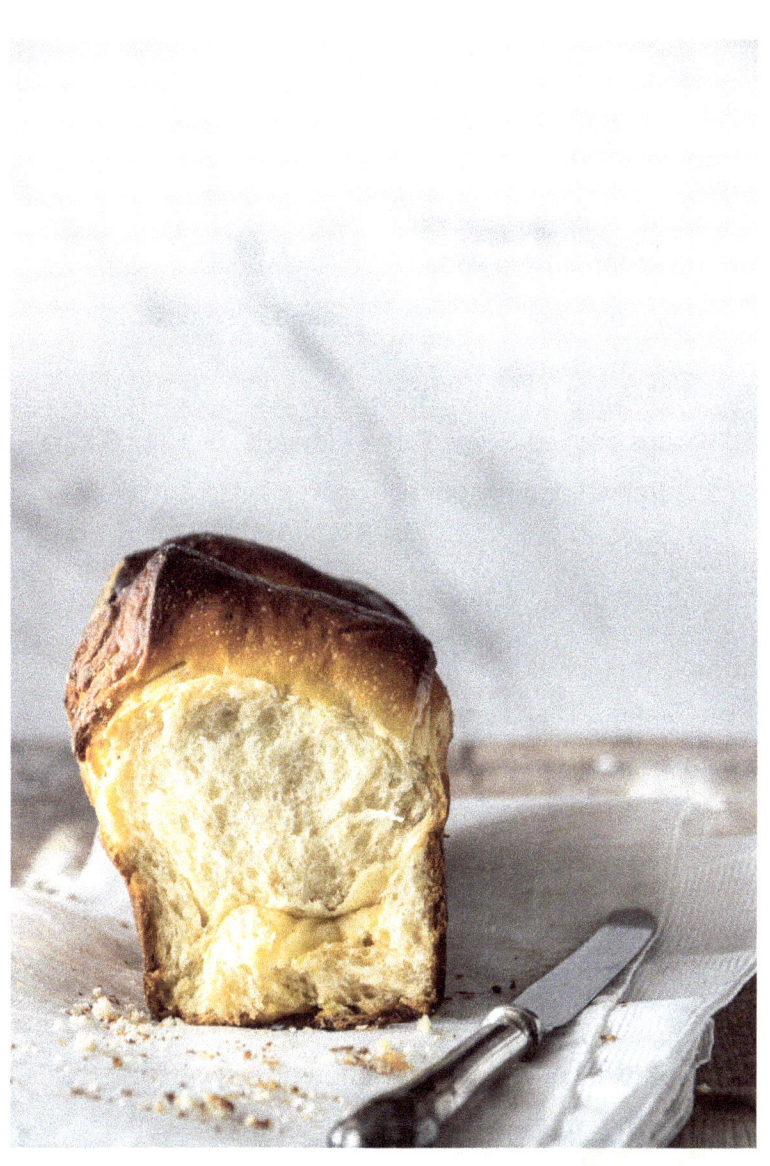

Tomato Sauce Bread

Dry Ingredients

- 1½ cups golden flaxseed meal
- ¼ teaspoon baking soda
- 1 teaspoon baking powder ½ teaspoon sea salt

Wet Ingredients

- 1¼ cups cooked Great Northern beans, or 1 (15.8-ounce) can, drained and rinsed
- 1 (8-ounce) can tomato sauce
- ⅓ cup liquid egg whites 1 teaspoon vinegar

Directions

1. Preheat the oven to 350°F.
2. Cover a 9 × 13-inch baking sheet with Pan Lining Paper, foil side down.
3. In a medium bowl, mix together the dry ingredients.
4. Blend wet ingredients thoroughly in blender.
5. Transfer the wet mixture to the bowl of dry ingredients. Mix well and quickly.
6. Scrape the batter onto the prepared baking sheet. Push the mixture to the edges, then level with a spatula. Bake for about 60 minutes or until dry to the touch.
7. Place upside down on a cooling rack. Remove the pan and paper. Let cool.
8. After cooling, cut into desired pieces or use as a prebaked pizza crust. Store in a sealed container in the refrigerator.

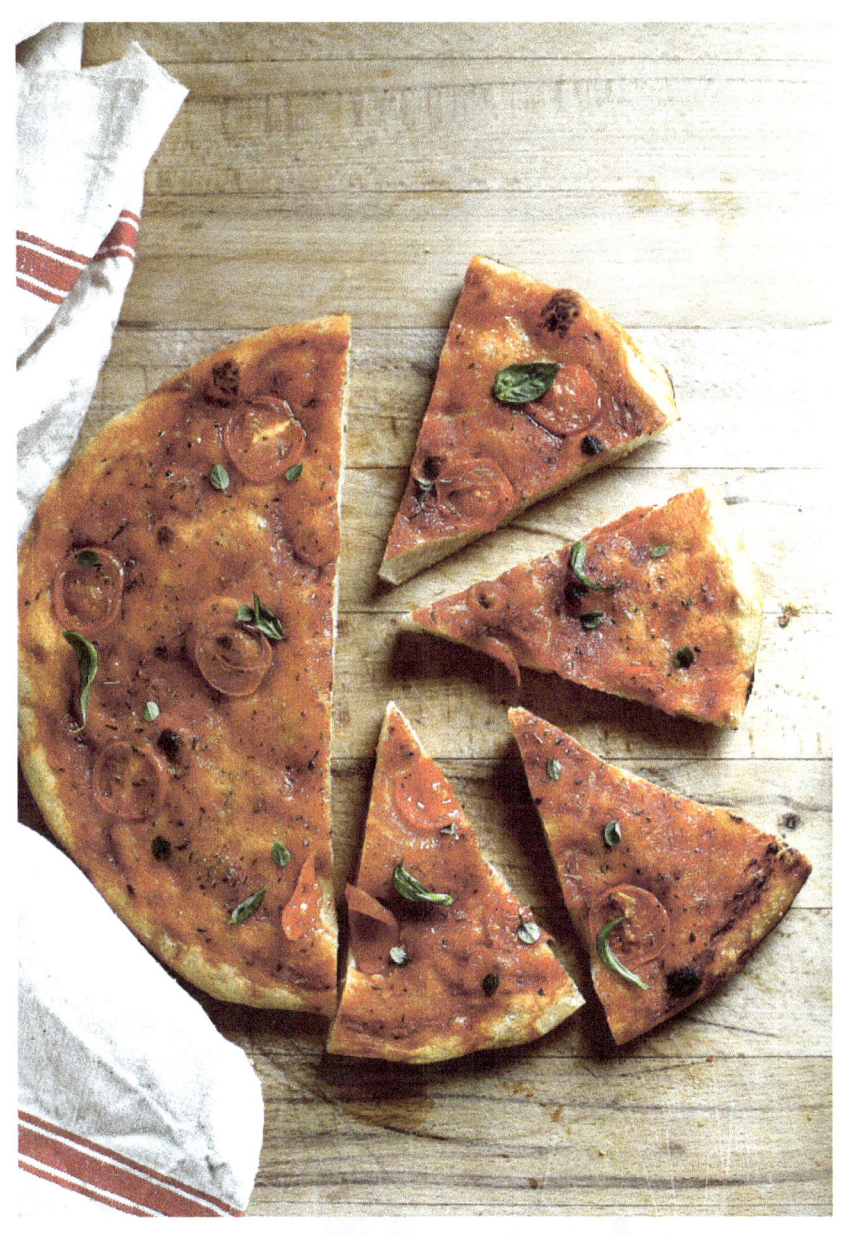

MEDITERRANEAN APPETIZERS

Mediterranean Nachos

Total time: 12 minutes

Prep time: 10 minutes

Cook time: 2 minutes

Yield: 6 servings

Ingredients

- 2 tsp. oil from jar of sun-dried tomatoes
- 2 tbsp. chopped sun-dried tomatoes in oil
- 2 tbsp. chopped Kalamata olives
- 1 tbsp. chopped green onion
- 1 small plum tomato, finely chopped
- 30 restaurant-style corn tortilla chips
- 1 (4 oz.) package crumbled feta cheese

Directions

- Mix together oil from the jar, sun-dried tomatoes, olives, onion, and plum tomato in a small bowl; set aside.
- Arrange the tortilla chips on a large microwavable plate and evenly top with cheese.
- Microwave on high for about 1 minute; rotate the plate and microwave for 1 minute more or until cheese is melted and bubbly.
- Evenly spoon the tomato mixture over the chips and cheese to serve.

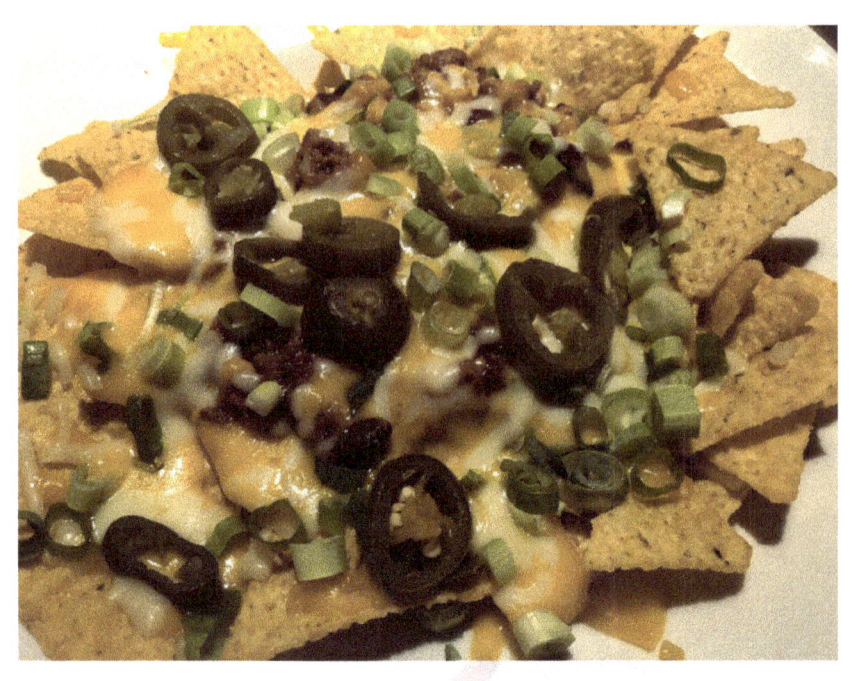

Roasted Beet Muhammara

Total time: 1 hour 20 minutes

Prep time: 20 minutes

Cook time: 1 hour

Yield: 1 ½ Cups

Ingredients

- 9 oz. trimmed and rinsed red beets
- ¼ cup plus 1 tbsp. extra virgin olive oil, divided
- 1 ½ tsp. freshly squeezed lemon juice
- 1 ½ tbsp. pomegranate molasses
- ½ cup sliced scallions
- 3/4 cup lightly toasted walnuts
- 1 tsp. ground cumin
- 1 tsp. Aleppo pepper
- Sea salt

Directions

- Place a rack in the center of oven and preheat to 375°F.
- Place beets in a baking dish and rub with 1 tablespoon extra virgin olive oil and cover with foil.
- Roast in the preheated oven for about 1 hour or until tender.
- Remove from oven and let cool; peel and then chop to yield 1 cup.
- In a food processor, pulse together the beets, scallions, and walnuts until finely chopped.

- Add lemon juice, pomegranate molasses, cumin, pepper, ½ teaspoon sea salt and the remaining extra virgin olive oil; process until very smooth. Adjust seasoning to your liking and serve cold or at room temperature.

www.ingramcontent.com/pod-product-compliance
Lightning Source LLC
Chambersburg PA
CBHW070032040426
42333CB00040B/1572